THE SELF-HYPNOSIS BOOK

This book is dedicated to the memory of Bill Atkinson-Ball, the first President of the Corporation of Advanced Hypnotherapy and founder of the Atkinson-Ball College of Hypnotherapy and HypnoHealing.
We pay tribute to him via this book for the knowledge, wisdom and inspiration that he gave to us, the authors, and to his hundreds of students of advanced hypnotherapy.

THE SELF-HYPNOSIS BOOK

CHERITH POWELL *and* GREG FORDE

VIKING
STUDIO

ADVICE TO THE READER

Before using this book and tape you are recommended to consult your doctor if you suffer from any dietary or health problems or special conditions, or are in any doubt.

VIKING STUDIO

Published by the Penguin Group
Penguin Putnam Inc.,
375 Hudson Street, New York, N.Y. 10014, U.S.A.
Penguin Books Ltd, 27 Wrights Lane,
London W8 5TZ, England
Penguin Books Australia Ltd, Ringwood,
Victoria, Australia
Penguin Books Canada Ltd, 10 Alcorn Avenue,
Toronto, Ontario, Canada M4V 3B2
Penguin Books (N.Z.) Ltd, 182–190 Wairau Road,
Auckland 10, New Zealand

Penguin Books Ltd, Registered Offices:
Harmondsworth, Middlesex, England

First published in the United States of America by Penguin Books 1996

20 19 18 17 16 15 14 13

An Eddison • Sadd Edition
Edited, designed and produced by
Eddison Sadd Editions Limited
St Chad's House, 148 King's Cross Road
London WC1X 9DH

CIP data available
ISBN 0-670-86530-3

Phototypeset in Berling using QuarkXpress on Apple Macintosh
Printed in China, produced by Phoenix Offset through The Hanway Press Ltd, UK

Contents

Introduction

When we started out to put this kit together we tried to imagine what kind of person would be interested in its contents. We asked ourselves a few questions to help us focus on why you, the reader, might want to use it. Could it be just idle curiosity? Doubtful—because you have already gone to the trouble to pick the kit up off the shelf and paid good money for it.

Is it because you feel driven to prove that this particular book is just another load of old baloney on the subject? Do you want to prove for yourself, once and for all, that hypnosis is all just rubbish? Possibly—because skeptics have been trying for centuries to do just that.

Is it because you have been influenced by a general interest in the subject of hypnosis? Probably—because increasing numbers of people do seem to have a fascination for both hypnosis and any kind of mind expanding technique.

Or is it because you have been feeling for some time that hypnosis could help you make positive changes in your life? This is more than likely—because ours seems to be an age when people are more questioning and, possibly, more open to personal growth and change.

Well, whatever your personal reasons, we welcome your interest and hope that we can answer some, if not all, of your questions. But, important as that may be, this kit is not just about answering questions. It is about action, and it is about taking action for yourself, at your own pace, and about discovering and using your own powers. Use this kit to unlock your own potential but do not be in too much of a rush. Prepare yourself. The most important step is for you to feel safe and secure. The next is to have the desire to use hypnosis. We aim to give you both.

Throughout the kit, you will find that we use images and everyday examples to illustrate our points. For example, we like to use the simple analogy of a motor car when discussing certain aspects of hypnosis. This analogy goes something like this:

The subconscious mind is like a preprogrammed, driverless motor car. It will automatically take the road that it knows and has no ability to steer itself or to deviate from its well-run route, or even to accelerate its progress. But by using self-hypnosis, you become the driver of that car. You can steer it in a new direction, you can show it how other routes might be more interesting or beneficial, you can show it all the other journeys it can make, now that YOU are the driver and now that YOU are in control.

By the time you have read this book and listened to the tape, you will have a choice. Your choice will be to remain "stuck" behind that preprogrammed car's steering wheel or to break free from some of those old, limiting beliefs. If this is a completely new concept in choice for you, view the following pages and the next few days as a period of transition because miracles do not happen overnight. Just remember that, sometimes, being "stuck" means being safe, so give yourself time.

You may well ask what all the fuss is about. As you probably know, hypnosis has been around for ages yet it is still shrouded in myth and mystique. Whenever people talk about hypnosis, the "experts" always seem to be on hand to expound upon its dangers. These can range from folklore about "your grandma wouldn't like it," to warnings about the hypnotist taking control of your mind or to the specter of devil worship.

This does not surprise us. Since the dawn of creation, humankind has instinctively feared the unknown. As a result, we have established myths and legends as a way of explaining what could not be understood. And hypnosis remains misunderstood. If this observation summons up the image of prehistoric man squatting at an open fire outside a cave dwelling, your starting point is probably only a few years too early.

Come forward a few steps in time to the nuclear age. When it comes to the subject of hypnosis, the average citizen of the modern era is still sitting outside the equivalent of that cave dwelling, perhaps even more deeply locked in a mental stone age than his prehistoric ancestor! Modern man is so often bound up with trivial concerns that he is unable to accept hypnosis, not only as a useful tool for making positive life changes but also as an essential element of survival. Through the pages of this book, we aim to undo that binding. We aim to show you that you have already been using some form of hypnosis every day of your life without knowing it.

That last statement might come as a shock. Modern man has believed his own press statements for so long that he is convinced of his super-intelligence and continually congratulates himself on his abilities: to travel into outer space with impunity; to tamper with basic building blocks of life through genetic engineering; to determine his own destiny even! So why is the idea that he can harness hypnosis so difficult to grasp?

Our own views begin with a fundamental recognition: most of us—and we, the authors, include ourselves in this—behave according to what we believe to be true. We call these our belief structures. And where do those belief structures come from? They were formed during our earliest years, while we were at the tender mercies of parents, siblings, teachers and even the media. And they are still being formed. The irony is that we are helping to reinforce them ourselves, day in, day out. In fact, most of our limiting beliefs belonged to someone else before we took them on board.

Maybe you recall the enchanting childhood story, "The Emperor's New Clothes?" The pompous, pampered old emperor and his servile courtiers all believed what they were told in order not to appear foolish or unfashionable. It is a good example of the power of suggestion and it illustrates only too well how we can all be programmed to believe something outrageous if the message is put across strongly enough. It also shows you that if you are not ready to take control of your own mind, someone else will quite happily do it for you. This realization may be all the encouragement you need to explore hypnosis.

Our hope is that, as you learn more about how the subconscious mind works, you will better understand why we behave in the ways we do and how certain messages become part of our everyday lives. Only then can you learn how to start substituting more suitable messages for those old, limiting ones.

Which brings us to the main aims of *The Self Hypnosis Kit*. We intend to dispel some of the myths surrounding hypnosis and show how you can use it for yourself. We will show you how hypnosis can be used both for deep relaxation and also as a means of empowerment. We will show how it can be used to form the basis for making positive beneficial changes and to reprogram old belief structures. Rest assured that, whatever you choose to use it for, you will really get to know yourself and your own potential in a way that you might never have envisioned.

The Self-Hypnosis Kit is designed for you to work with on an individual basis, at a level that feels safe and secure for you. So if you are not ready to consider taking full responsibility for yourself, do not worry. Use the kit to grow in confidence and self-esteem until you find your own safe and secure level. But if you do feel ready, right now, to break free from those negative programs of the past, then this kit will give you the ability to realize your full potential and start making those beneficial changes. We believe our combination of book and audio tape is a powerful one that will allow you, the reader and listener, to enter into self-hypnosis within a few days. The only really satisfactory way to learn self-hypnosis is when you are already in hypnosis. That is why a hypnotic tape is supplied with this book.

We also firmly believe that there is no limit to the value of hypnosis. The only limitations are within your mind. So just in case you did not get the message the first time (modern man and modern woman can be obstinate when it comes to making changes), we reiterate that your mind is there to serve you, not to rule you. If you opt to break free from some of those old, limiting beliefs you can begin to accept responsibility for yourself while at the same time letting others accept responsibility for themselves. Regard your journey as the retrieval of something that goes back to the very beginning of time—our natural birthright, our ability to connect to our inner resources and use them to the full. We are privileged to be your travelling companions.

Important Notice

We urge you NOT to play the audio tape until you have read through to Chapter Four. If you hold off playing the tape until that stage, what you have read will make better sense and what you hear will be more powerful. You will be both better equipped and more eager to go forward into Chapters Five and Six where you will discover how to enhance your new-found skills.

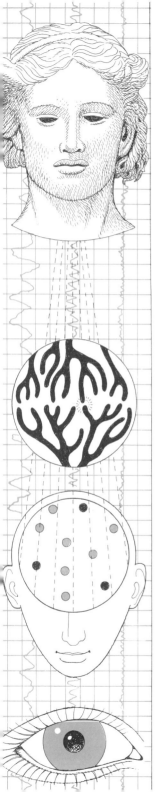

Chapter One

Hypnosis: the Truth

If we were to say, right here and now, that everyone goes into hypnosis naturally every day of their lives, very few people would believe us. Until, that is, we explain that hypnosis is really just a day-dreaming state. Most of us can acknowledge that we day-dream on a fairly regular basis. Even those people who claim that they never day-dream do, in fact, go through a state of hypnosis twice a day. The first occasion is just prior to waking in the morning (a "hypnagogic" state), and the second is just before going to sleep at night (a "hypnopompic" state).

But do not let that confuse you. There are almost as many definitions of the word "hypnosis" as there are types of hypnotherapy, and every dictionary you pick up will have a different definition.

The word itself comes from the Ancient Greek, *Hypnos* (top left), who was the god of sleep. So, is hypnosis another form of sleep? Well, not quite. It is neither being asleep nor being fully awake, but could perhaps be described as feeling sleepy, yet at the same time being hyper-aware. *Now* are you feeling confused? Read on.

Everyman's Encyclopedia defines hypnosis as, "...a condition of artificially induced sleep." However, when a person is asleep, they are oblivious to all that is going on around them. If someone spoke to you quietly when you were asleep, the chances are that you would not hear them, nor would you remember anything of what they had said. In no way would you be in control of the situation. Hypnosis is not at all like that.

M.J. Bass, writing in the *Journal of Experimental Psychology* in 1931, proved conclusively that there is a difference between hypnosis and sleep. In laboratory tests he found that the patellar reflex—the knee-jerk reaction—of patients in hypnosis was exactly the same as when they were in their waking state. During sleep, there was virtually no response at all.

The *Encyclopaedia Britannica* is closer to the mark and fairer. It likens hypnosis to sleep, but only superficially, for it claims that the subject in hypnosis is in a special psychological state characterized by a receptiveness and responsiveness more attuned than would be the case in the ordinary conscious state.

The Soviet physiologist, Ivan Pavlov, said that the hypnotic state is a "partial sleep," understanding it as a state of sleep in which a "point of vigilance" persists in the cerebral cortex. He also said that ,"Hypnosis is nothing but the manifestation of an emotional state of increased intensity."

Power to Refuse
Is hypnosis brainwashing in disguise?

This is another popular misconception, perhaps reinforced by stage hypnosis shows where viewers believe that the subject is being told what to do and has no power to refuse. Many experiments in brainwashing were conducted during the Second World War, and it was found that it was impossible to brainwash someone without the use of drugs. Because of the potential for carrying out covert operations through brainwashing without putting their own agents at risk, both the Western and Eastern Blocs engaged in in-depth research on hypnosis over a number of years. They found that, in order to achieve the desired results, they not only had to change the subject's perception of his world, but physically had to change his world. This was accomplished by imprisonment, sensory deprivation and drugs.

Ernest Hilgard, author of *Divided Consciousness* (1977) states that, "Hypnotism is merely a state of high suggestibility—it is not gullibility." An ethical hypnotherapist should only be concerned with the client's well-being, and will therefore only make suggestions which are for the client's benefit. But, even if that were not the case, Hilgard's assertions (confirming earlier experiments conducted by others) claimed that the hypnotized subject could not be induced to harm themselves or to become anti-social. He found that hypnosis and hypnotherapy could be carried out only with the co-operation of the patient. Hypnosis is truly a consent state.

A related theory was that brain fatigue takes place because of the monotonous repetition of suggestions by the hypnotists. This can be discounted immediately in view of the fact that a good hypnotherapist can induce hypnosis in a matter of seconds.

Hypnosis and Meditation
Is there a difference between the two?

Ormond McGill, known in America as "The Dean of Hypnosis," has spent years studying hypnosis and meditation, and he maintains that hypnosis is not meditation, but is, in fact, just the opposite. According to him, the motivation behind hypnosis is to achieve a given goal, whereas meditation is non-motivated and has no goal to achieve. He goes on to say, "Hypnosis is best understood by regarding it as a way of instructing the mind or programming the mind, so it will affect the autonomic nervous system rather than the sympathetic nervous system, as is most noticeably the case in everyday behaviour."

Medical Theories
Doctors and therapists attempt to describe hypnosis from a medical perspective

James Braid (pages 23 to 24), the pioneering Scottish doctor who first coined the word "hypnosis," established that it was, "an altered state of consciousness," where the patient is deeply relaxed, and yet at the same time fully alert.

John Hartland, an American physician and hypnotherapist, has said that, "Most people agree that hypnosis can loosely be defined as a state of mind in which suggestions are not only more readily accepted than in the waking state, but are also acted upon much more powerfully."

Dr. Fred Frankel, Professor of Psychiatry at Harvard Medical School, once stated: "Clinicians learn readily that they exercise control over most patients only to the extent that the patients are prepared to let them, which leads to the often expressed opinion, 'all hypnosis is self-hypnosis.'"

In their book, *Clinical Hypnotherapy*, David Cheek and Leslie LeCron define hypnosis as "A state of having increased suggestibility, literalness of understanding and willingness to comply with optimistic suggestions."

Sigmund Freud's early use of hypnosis led him to advance the theory—argued by others—that hypnosis gives access to a less sophisticated part of the mind. Freud went on to claim that if a person could be easily hypnotized, that person was psychologically healthy.

Of course, there are some people who theorize that there is no such thing as hypnosis, and that certain people either act in that way to please the hypnotist or are just role-playing. One major skeptic, the American psychologist, Theodore Barber, has consistently claimed that there is no such thing as hypnosis, and that people can do the same things when given "task-motivating" instructions in the normal wakeful state.

As Doctor James Esdaile (page 24) must have thought in the 1800s, it is truly amazing that someone can pretend not to feel pain, especially when having an arm or a leg amputated!

Scientific Proof

Recent quantitative research, under laboratory conditions, confirm the beliefs of the early pioneers

Investigations in America during the early 1970s sought to measure the electrical changes that occur in the brain during hypnosis. Results of these investigations proved that hypnosis did alter the brain wave patterns and also the chemistry of the nervous system.

Research carried out in the former Soviet Union also established definite changes, both physical and psychological, during hypnosis. The use of electronic equipment proved that it was a "state" which was different to both sleep and being awake.

Recent scientific applications have given us further confirmation—through recording techniques such as biofeedback—that definite physiological changes take place when a subject is in hypnosis. In the deeply relaxed state of hypnosis, the parasympathetic nervous system—a sort of subconscious nervous system we will discuss further in Chapter Five—is switched on. As a result, breathing slows down, the heart beats slower, and all the muscles in the body become profoundly relaxed. Another signal that a patient is in hypnosis is the appearance of rapid eye movements (REMS)—a rapid, fluttering action, also associated with deep sleep, which is certainly something that cannot be faked.

The experiments with electroencephalograms (EEG) by such people as Professor Wyke at The Royal College of Surgeons in London and by Professor Ulett at the American Psychiatric Association again showed that there are definite changes in the electrical activity of the brain when a client is in hypnosis.

Because it induced such deep physical relaxation, some scientists, such as Morton Prince and Ivan Pavlov, claimed that the hypnotic state was characterized by, "various partial dissociations of awareness." Again, this is questionable, bearing in mind what the eminent American hypnotherapist, Dave Elman claims: "A client in hypnosis can be two thousand times more aware than when he is in the conscious state." Elman explained this statement to a group of doctors by reminding them of a regression which he had just carried out on a young lady, where she had "re-lived" the first day that she had walked. She was fully aware of everything around her, the details of the furniture in the room, the yellow dress that she was wearing, the print dress with colors that her mother was wearing, and most interesting of all, the feelings that she had as that one-year-old child.

Obviously the majority of people would have no recall at all of such an event, although we know that it happened to all of us at one time, but in hypnosis all those early memories, complete to the tiniest detail, can be retrieved in glorious technicolor.

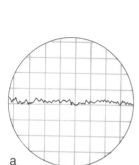

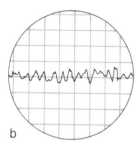

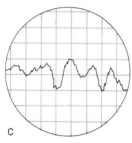

Electroencephalograms illustrating electrical activity in the brain: while wide awake (a), in light hypnosis (b), and in deep hypnosis (c).

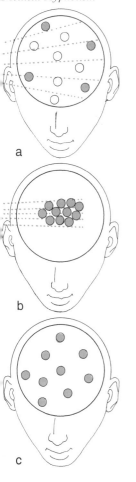

Units of mind power are scattered throughout the brain. In an ordinary state, only a few units are affected by suggestion (a). In hypnosis, the units are focused together and all are affected (b). After hypnosis, the units are scattered once more but each one now carries a dose of the suggestion (c). Source: *British Journal of Medical Hypnotism*

a

b

c

So, what is hypnosis? Is it a "condition" or "a state of mind?" Dave Elman challenges the word "condition," pointing out that it implies a persisting quality, being slow to change. A "state," he maintains, is transient, more analogous to a mood, changing easily and frequently. As a result, he describes hypnosis as being "a state of mind."

A good illustration of what many believe happens to the mind before, during, and after hypnosis is shown on this page. Scattered randomly throughout the brain are what are termed "units of mind power." Under hypnosis, these units are focused together and all are able to receive a suggestion. After hypnosis, the units disperse once again but each one now carries elements of what was suggested.

By now you have probably had enough of the various theories. But hypnosis is hard to pin down and we must admit that sometimes it is easier to explain what hypnosis is not, rather than what it is. Hypnosis is not sleep. It is not a state of being unconscious. It is not going into a coma, nor even a feeling of drifting off into outer space!

While consciousness is entirely suspended in natural sleep, it is most definitely present in hypnosis. This, of course, makes all the difference. In hypnosis, the subject is aware of everything that is going on around them, and can remember everything afterwards. Even if a hypnotherapist were to give a client a post-hypnotic suggestion to the effect that the client would have absolutely no recollection of the session, the information would in fact return to the client's consciousness within a relatively short period of time, usually beginning with the periods just prior to, and just after sleep.

Most hypnotherapists would agree that any hypnosis is self-hypnosis, inasmuch as it has to be a state of co-operation. In other words, no one can be hypnotized unless they actively wish to enter the state of hypnosis. So an ethical hypnotherapist will realize that he or she is merely acting as a catalyst, as a facilitator, to help clients to help themselves.

We believe that everybody enters hypnosis every day, naturally, but is unaware of doing so—perhaps while listening to music, day-dreaming or routinely washing dishes. We also believe that anybody can learn to enter that state voluntarily and use it for their benefit. We say that hypnosis is the state of being deeply relaxed but, at the same time, engaged, alert, focused and fully aware of what is going on.

The Hypnotized Subject's Response

Ordinary people who have undergone hypnosis attempt to describe the experience

We have asked clients how they feel when they are in the state we call hypnosis. We have found that their feedback ranges from feelings of lethargy to surprise at being fully aware, of being able to hear everything around them with almost pinpoint accuracy, and, most important of all, of knowing that they were in control at all times. Along with the general feeling of lethargy, many clients feel somewhat detached and their eyelids get heavy and want to close. Some clients may want to follow the suggestions given by the hypnotherapist, others may not. What is most certainly obvious to the client is that they are completely in control, maintain all their mental faculties, and are in no way unconscious nor deeply asleep.

In fact, on their first session, most people are disappointed to experience just how ordinary hypnosis is and how unlike the magical or mystical state that they had been led to expect. All too often it feels entirely natural. Which is exactly what it is.

Some recent remarks which spring to mind include the following.

• *"I used my self-hypnosis when I went to the dentist, and didn't need any anesthesia at all. The dentist was amazed."*

• *"I used my trigger in the supermarket where I always have panic attacks. This time it just didn't happen. I actually got all my shopping and went through the check-out just like a normal person. What a relief!"*

• *"I feel it is no exaggeration to say that self-hypnosis has changed, if not saved, my life. For the first time in years I really feel good about myself."*

• *"It is three years since I saw you as a client, but I have always practiced my self-hypnosis on a regular basis. Recently I had an accident on my motorcycle, breaking my leg in three places. I remembered what you had said about mind and body healing themselves, so I worked on my leg from the inside to help knit the bones together quickly. My surgeon has told me that the fractures have healed in about half the time that he would have expected—fantastic!"*

• *"I haven't felt so good in months and people have commented on how much better I look—I've woken up. As a social worker and mother what you taught me was the missing piece of a jigsaw puzzle."*

• *"I used my self-hypnosis to stop smoking and surprise, surprise, after so many attempts in the past, I've finally done it. I have been free of cigarettes now for over two months and there were absolutely no withdrawal symptoms at all."*

• *"After just 12 days of using self-hypnosis, the pain in my left side has disappeared and I have experienced no recurrence of it since. This is truly amazing, as I did not believe the pain would ever go away, despite all the previous medical treatment I had received. This has made me realize just how effective hypnosis is."*

The list could go on almost indefinitely—we have just taken the above examples at random from some of the letters received from our clients and students of our self-hypnosis classes.

Tying the Threads Together

We attempt to draw together all the many observations and assertions

An inspirational essay on hypnotism was written by William Wesley Cook MD at the turn of the century. At that time, Cook was Professor of Physiological Medicine at the University of Chicago. We believe that so much of what he said then remains pertinent today.

"Hypnotism is the most practical science of the age. It enters into our everyday life, and confers advantages that cannot be acquired through any other medium. Its practice is no longer a mere pastime for amusement and sensation, as professional persons of the highest standing now recognize its value and seek to profit by its benefits. Scientists regard it as a natural power, for ages kept dormant, but apparently destined to perform an active part in the welfare and development of future generations.

"It does not require years of study to become a hypnotist, for this great blessing to humanity is a natural endowment possessed by practically everyone and capable of being developed by all who will devote to its study the patience and energy always so necessary for the development of natural talents.

"The practical ability of the science of hypnotism is universally recognized. Thousands are eagerly seeking to learn its principles and laws, that they may reap the benefits of its powers.

"Prejudice, bigotry, and narrow-minded sophistry have until lately succeeded in smothering the great science of hypnotism. Those who were bold enough to make known the marvellous nature of the hypnotic power they were able to manifest, were denounced as wizards, charlatans, imposters and mountebanks. But now the tables have turned. Those who were formerly denounced are now regarded as scientific investigators, and the doctrines they taught are being eagerly learned by the most noted scientists. What was held up for ridicule is now regarded as a dignified science. What was attributed to evil machinations is now regarded as one of the greatest blessings to the human race.

"Hypnotism has triumphed. It occupies the position of a dignified science, and with its present impetus and its future certainty of development, it is destined to startle the world by its marvellous revelations."

Written some ninety years ago, we imagine that Doctor Cook would be disappointed that hypnotism has not achieved quite the recognition that he envisioned but, certainly, progress has been made.

The fact that there is no generally accepted definition of the word hypnosis and its many uses may be an advantage, as it places no limits on our views, uses and explorations of hypnosis in personal or therapeutic situations. Nor does it limit the help that it can be in improving the quality of someone's life. A simple conclusion therefore might be to describe hypnosis as an aid to finding answers that you already know, but did not know you know, and then being able to consider the information and learn from it to the extent that you can modify your behavior.

So, where does all this leave you in your query as to what you personally might expect hypnosis to be? All we can say is that only experimentation with this book and tape will give you the answer, because each individual has a very personal experience in hypnosis.

We can, however, promise you one thing—if you read the book, listen to the tape and practice your self-hypnosis on a regular basis, following our guidelines, the quality of your life will improve enormously. What more can you ask?

We hope we have whetted your appetite and that now you are wondering about the history of the hypnotic skills you are about to learn. It might help you on your own journey if we first took you back in time to review the background of hypnosis. A sage once said, "There is absolutely nothing new on this earth," and that is certainly true of hypnosis. If we told you that hypnosis goes back about four thousand years, we would not be exaggerating.

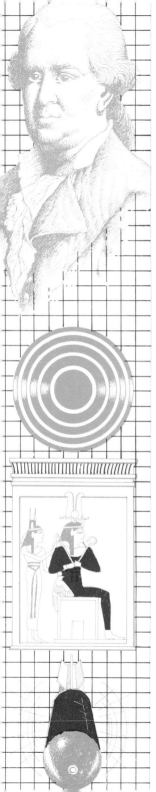

Chapter Two

Hypnosis Through the Ages

Imagine that you live in Ancient Egypt. Imagine that you have some kind of mental, emotional or physical problem. Now, you have a decision to make. Do you drop into your local pharmacy to get some magic pills to make you better? Or do you go to your local doctor and sit alongside other sick people in the waiting room until it is your turn? No, you do not. You get into your own personal chariot and take yourself to the equivalent of a modern health farm: you pay a visit to one of the Egyptian "sleep temples." There, you stay for one month, in a trance-like state and wait to get better. The Ancient Egyptians knew what many of our modern doctors fail to remember, and that is that mind and body in unison can heal themselves, given adequate rest. The hypnosis the Ancient Egyptians used shut out self-inflicted babble from their conscious minds to facilitate healing.

But maybe you do not live in Egypt. So let us try Ancient Greece where they have "healing shrines" that work on the same principle as the sleep temples in Egypt. Now we are also getting closer to home, because, as we have already said, the word hypnosis originates from the Greek word for sleep.

Of course, in these ancient times, it helps if you are religious. Hypnosis seemed to play a major part in religious rites practiced by the clergy, and archeologists have found many engravings showing worshippers who were undoubtedly in some sort of trance. One such engraving shows Chiron, a well known Ancient Greek physician, placing one of his patients into hypnosis in preparation for an operation. Both oracles and physicians of that time used either hypnosis, narcotic herbs or pungent volcanic fumes! Take your pick—we certainly know which one we would prefer.

Our time travels also prove that it is no new

concept that the mind affects the body. As far back as 350 BC Hippocrates, known as "the father of medicine," stated that all feelings and emotions start in the brain, and that those feelings and emotions are the source of any disease in the body. Hippocrates reasoned that if you can influence the brain, you can influence the body. So, if you are living in Greece at this time you might get the chance to attend the Medical School and Guild founded by Hippocrates on the Aegean island of Cos, and you might even get the chance to read one or more of the seventy impressive volumes that he wrote, known as the *Hippocratic Corpus*. There you would find the very beginnings of the search to find the connection between mind and body.

Such ideas regarding the mind-body connection were held by Indian mystics (yogis), by tribal shamans in Africa, the Americas and Antipodes, and a broad spectrum of people all over the globe. Innumerable documents, paintings, and engravings found in every corner of the world illustrate the fact that hypnosis has been widely practiced for centuries. In these cultures, feats of healing were invariably linked with a hypnotic ceremony or trance-inducing ritual that prepared the subject for the desired outcome. The process hinged on the subject's belief that the medicine man or shaman would work magic that could effect a cure.

For several centuries, hypnosis fell out of favor in Europe. This was probably due in no small part to the powerful influence of various religions, the leaders of which were after all employing their own form of hypnosis to control the masses. It resurfaced in Europe in the eighteenth century. It is, perhaps, no coincidence that this was a time when a great many people were becoming disenchanted with physicians and more than just a few doctors moved away from orthodox medicine in an attempt to find a universal cure for all ills.

Planets and Animal Magnetism
The early days of scientific study into hypnosis

Moving forward in our imaginary hypnosis-scanning time machine to eighteenth century Austria, we meet Franz Anton Mesmer (1734-1815), one of the earliest scientists to take a serious interest in hypnosis (shown at the top left of page 20). Mesmer started his career studying theology and medicine in Germany and at Vienna University, passing his exams with honours. It is interesting to note that his thesis was entitled *The Influence of the Planets on the Human Body*. Mesmer's early theory was that there were physical forces in the universe that exercise an unseen influence on the human body. This spooky idea was not terribly well received in some quarters! However, his theory gained ground a few years later when he met a Jesuit priest, Maximillian Hell, who had been achieving miraculous results with disturbed ("hysterical") patients by applying magnets to their bodies. Perhaps, the two of them reasoned, the planetary influence was also a magnetic one.

Mesmer subsequently revised his earlier theories to claim that the planets affected the human organism through an invisible fluid, and that this fluid could be derived from magnets. He became convinced that there was a healing and magnetic power emanating from his own body and hands. This, he believed, was an entirely natural phenomenon. Thus he developed his theories of "animal magnetism," or what is now referred to as "mesmerism."

Initially, Mesmer seemed to effect dramatic cures. His methods were theatrical, as his treatments took place in a large darkened hall and all his patients sat around the outside of an oak tub which was filled with water. Into the water were placed strange objects such as iron filings, empty bottles, even broken glass. On top of the tub was placed a wooden cover pierced with iron rods. The patients held these rods or applied them to the diseased parts of their bodies.

Ostracized by the medical fraternity, then ordered to leave Vienna, Mesmer met his downfall after moving to Paris, when he often made dangerously incorrect diagnoses that led to him being widely discredited. Mesmerism was further set back by a commission set up in France to examine the phenomenon. Headed by Benjamin Franklin (the American Ambassador in France at that time), the commission totally discredited the effectiveness of mesmerism, attributing Mesmer's many cures to some as yet unknown physiological cause. Sadly, Mesmer and his colleagues could not grasp the psychological implications of animal magnetism and were too early to foresee the therapeutic benefits derived from either autosuggestion or hypnosis. Yet his experiments and successes led the way for others.

Ironically, recent research in the area of quantum physics suggests mesmerism has some validity, the theory being that electromagnetism (not animal magnetism) has a definite effect on chemical reactions within the body.

First Steps into Hypnosis
Pioneering attitudes lead the way

Moving forward in time, we could stop our machine a little later in the eighteenth century and travel to Scotland to meet Doctor James Braid. Braid rejected the idea of animal magnetism and proved conclusively that no fluid passed from healer to patient. He suggested that the mesmeric state was just a form of sleep. Classically educated, Braid was the first person to coin the word "hypnosis." Braid started out skeptical but his experiments did away with many myths and he demonstrated success when dealing with incurable illnesses or conditions labelled "nervous complaints." His experiments also proved that when a subject was in hypnosis, his personal integrity was even more secure than when he was in the fully awake state—he showed that the subject is not without will nor is he under the will of the hypnotist. Braid's subjects could not be forced to do things against their will and his controlled studies were the first to show that the relationship between subject and hypnotist was based upon co-operation and reason.

It was also Braid who showed that hypnosis could be induced simply by the patient fixing his eyes on a single object (which is still the basis of most hypnotic inductions to this day). Spurred on by his successes, he became so convinced of its therapeutic use that he advocated the more general use of hypnotism to alleviate anxiety and pain.

Thanks to Braid, hypnosis emerged as a "new science" and, after violent opposition and against all odds, gained respectability, albeit temporarily.

Hypnotic Anesthesia
"God intended people to suffer"

Moving forward again to the mid-1800s, we travel to Calcutta in India to meet another Scottish doctor, James Esdaile. There, Esdaile performed over three thousand operations using only hypnosis as an anesthetic. More than three hundred of them were for major surgery. At that time the mortality rate following operations ranged between twenty-five and fifty per cent. However, when Esdaile started using hypnotic anesthesia, he was delighted to find that his fatalities dropped to only five per cent. He did not know why this phenomenon occurred. Present day knowledge could lead to the assumption that the subconscious mind develops a greater resistance to infection when hypnosis is used.

Sadly, Esdaile did not succeed in convincing his more conventional colleagues of the effectiveness of hypnosis as they maintained that his patients were just pretending they could not feel any pain to please him! Brought to trial by the British Medical Association, Esdaile finally lost his licence. It was stated at the trial that he was blasphemous for even attempting to control pain and it was publicly declared that "God intended people to suffer."

We hope you are not getting tired with all this travelling around but it gets even more exciting as we move on in time and into Europe. To Paris, to be precise, to consult with a Doctor Jean Martin Charcot. Charcot was a neurologist and professor of diseases of the nervous system, and he demonstrated that many hysterical or obscure symptoms could be reduced or even removed by hypnosis. An interesting part of his work was to prove that it was not only women who suffered from hysteria. Up to that time, it had been assumed that hysteria was caused by a displaced womb (taken from the Greek word *hustera* for uterus). Charcot pursued Mesmer's ideas of animal magnetism but his most important contribution was to stimulate an interest in the psychological causes of hysteria and the use of hypnosis in treating it. In so doing, he attracted the attention of one of the most outstanding figures of the twentieth century.

The Dawn of Psychoanalysis
The role of hypnosis in developing an understanding of the human psyche

We still have not quite reached the twentieth century, but we are almost there as we return to Austria. If you are rich, and living in Vienna, you are likely to meet Sigmund Freud, about whom enough books have been written to fill a modest library.

Freud first practiced medicine in Vienna, specializing in neurology, and in 1885 he moved to Paris where he studied under Jean Charcot. He later returned to Vienna and developed an interest in psychopathology. He was particularly struck by the success of curing hysteria by getting the patient to recollect, under hypnosis, the root origins of and the emotions associated with the hysteria. Freud and his growing band of followers believed that hypnosis was one avenue into the subconscious mind and that dream analysis was another. In his earliest attempts at psychoanalysis, he used hypnosis to uncover the subconscious roots of patients' problems and to recall traumatic experiences from childhood. Freud believed that by revealing a cause, a patient opened up a way to effect a cure.

Freud was among the first to develop the analytical techniques which we now know as psychoanalysis.

His use of hypnotic catharsis—a release of emotions under hypnosis—was later replaced by "free association" and "transference" on to the therapist. At first, Freud maintained that his psychotherapeutic technique could only be properly utilized with the use of hypnosis. However, he later abandoned this idea for two possible reasons. It is believed that Freud had difficulty looking people in the eye and therefore chose the easier option of sitting behind his clients as they lay on a couch. It is also said that he thought that some patients were recalling childhood fantasies rather than actual events. Whatever the precise reasons, Freud's rejection was a serious setback for hypnosis, given his enormous influence and following.

Carl Jung, an early colleague of Freud's, also had misgivings about hypnosis, but his theory regarding "the collective unconscious" opened up many avenues of research which still fascinate people today. Both Freud's and Jung's work depended very much on long term therapy and work with the individual unconcious—concepts that have been carried forward to the point where people often retain the services of their own personal analyst for many, many years. It would seem to us that an effective way of tuning into one's unconscious would surely be via hypnosis thereby resolving problems rapidly and dynamically.

At the beginning of the twentieth century, the British Medical Association investigated the medical application of hypnosis. They disapproved of it fully, possibly because of the proliferation of stage hypnosis shows at that time.

However, with the onset of the First World War, a large number of troops experienced a form of trance in battle, sometimes resulting in full paralysis. Because the medical profession had dismissed the theory of hysteria, the term "shell-shock" was coined. It was only after a number of men had been court-martialed and shot as cowards that it was realized that this state occurs naturally in the wild, when animals become rigid in order to avoid detection. Because this was happening subconsciously, it was found that hypnosis was an effective way of dealing with the syndrome. Hypnosis also gained credibility during the Second World War. In Japanese prisoner of war camps, the absence of chemical anesthetics resulted in some operations being carried out using hypnosis as the only form of pain control.

Developing the Art and Science of Hypnosis
British and American medical associations approve the use of hypnosis

Using our time machine after the Second World War, we travel to Australia in the 1950s and catch up with Ainslie Meares, an Australian psychiatrist. Meares developed a new train of thought, based on the theories of the Russian physiologist Ivan Pavlov, whereby in hypnosis the more sophisticated part of the brain was switched off, thus allowing for increased activity of the more primitive areas—what we know as the subconscious part of the mind.

Meares maintained that when a person was in hypnosis, the primitive areas of the mind were more open to suggestion. He argued that ideas were more readily accepted when freed from the logical criticism of the conscious mind, but also that they were more profoundly held.

But time is moving fast now, and we are on our travels again, this time to the United States of America to meet up with Doctor Milton Erickson, who had degrees both in medicine and psychology. He was the founding president of the American Society of Clinical Hypnosis.

Erickson was a major influence in the field of hypnotherapy because his approach was radically different. He adopted a much more permissive style compared to the rather authoritarian stance taken by previous hypnotists. His aim was to create a form of hypnosis based on a client's own lifestyle and interests, thereby causing his conscious mind to feel comfortable with the hypnotic state and enabling him to understand himself in a new way. His attitude was that the client should not be dominated by the therapist but should be encouraged to accept hypnosis as a totally natural state of mind and one that could be used to help the client to help himself.

Still in America, we also come across Dave Elman. Totally different in approach to Milton Erickson, Elman gave many dynamic presentations of how speedily and effectively hypnosis could be used in a wide range of therapies. His interest in hypnosis had begun when he was a boy of eight. Over a period of months, he watched his father dying slowly and very painfully with cancer. Doctors had said there was nothing they could do to relieve his father's suffering when one day a stage hypnotist came to the house and, from that moment on, after just a few minutes of hypnosis, the pain vanished. Dave Elman never forgot how his father was given relief in this way.

Elman worked first of all as a stage hypnotist, thereby developing the rapid induction techniques that became his trademark. He had no scientific training whatsoever, but at the age of 49, and at the request of doctors, he developed the Dave Elman Course in Clinical Hypnosis. He became known as one of the very best and most successful teachers of hypnosis in America.

Some of Elman's qualities, which the authors of this book have endeavored to emulate, were his use of rapid induction techniques, semantics, voice inflection, and his ability to create a positive expectation of change. His contribution made a huge step forward in the history of hypnosis, taking away much of the mystique surrounding the word itself, and really modernizing hypnotherapy for the twentieth century.

Another therapist, who adopted a more permissive approach like Milton Erickson, was an American lady, Virginia Satir. Her technique was such that her clients would hardly recognize the fact that they were in hypnosis. Her contributions to hypnotherapy included her work now widely known as "Family

Therapy." This was based on her experience of teaching handicapped children which led her to observe the behavior of the whole family and the interaction among family members.

Satir also developed a technique called "Parts Therapy," which is based on the assumption that our minds are made up of many different parts all dealing with different aspects of our personality. This has really formed the basis of more advanced techniques in hypnotherapy today.

We have been stuck in our time machine in America for rather a while now with the last three therapists, and we stay there just a little bit longer to look at the founders of Neuro-Linguistic Programming (NLP). We will give just a brief mention of it here because we will be going into detail about this later on in the book.

NLP was devised by Richard Bandler (a mathematician) and John Grinder (a linguist) and is comprised of a revolutionary package of techniques, based mostly on the work of their fellow Americans, Erickson and Satir. NLP has spawned considerable recent interest in the creation of models of human excellence in therapeutic fields as well as in industry, sports and so on. The use of NLP techniques in hypnosis has greatly advanced hypnotherapy.

All these later practitioners recognized one strikingly simple fact about hypnosis that we will have cause to reiterate many times throughout this book. Despite its checkered history, hypnosis is a completely natural state of mind, a state of mind that one enters spontaneously several times a day. As such, it is not always easy to know when one is actually in hypnosis. These later practitioners acknowledged its profoundly natural condition, and sought to find ways to harness it for the benefit of the individual. We like to think that, in this book, we take it up where they left off.

Finally, we must look at the work of Bill Atkinson-

Ball, the founder of the Atkinson-Ball College of Hypnotherapy and HypnoHealing in the United Kingdom, without whose work this book could not have been written. His innovative and inspiring work has done much to improve the standards of hypnotherapy in Britain and the United States. His rapid inductions and his intuition when dealing with clients were without equal. His research into hypnosis started at the University of Nottingham, England, where he had been sent by the Royal Air Force to study how hypnotic techniques could be used to help shell-shocked troops returning from Korea. He later used those techniques on himself to bring about a complete recovery from the arthritis resulting from an aerial accident. It was from that work that he developed his speciality, HypnoHealing. More of this later.

So, there we have it: a journey through the ages to look at the way hypnosis has developed over the centuries and how this development has contributed to the use of hypnosis for personal fulfillment. It might be appropriate to point out here that the present acceptance and recognition of hypnosis has taken a long time to evolve. Hypnosis has survived as a technique over the last few centuries because of the work of lay hypnotherapists, even theatrical hypnotists, who have kept it in the public eye and have in no small measure helped to spawn the huge interest in all the mind-expanding techniques used today.

Hypnosis or Not
A skeptic tries to prove that hypnosis does not exist

There are certain people, many of them psychologists, who busily try to prove that there is no such thing as hypnosis. Recently, on national television in Britain, a psychologist set about trying to prove that the hypnotic trance did not exist. He started out with the message that the trance state of hypnosis could not conclusively be proven to exist and, therefore, must be attributed to something else. He then conducted an hypnotic induction with a class of students who later stated, to a person, that as they were aware of everything that had occurred and could remember all that was said this could not have been hypnosis.

Some time later, the psychologist had a single student "pretend" to be in hypnosis. This student then began to exhibit some of the best outward signs of good-quality hypnosis, even though he was convinced that he was only acting. At one point, the psychologist achieved what is called full body catalepsy, or suspended animation, with the student. This is a condition where the body becomes so rigid that it can be propped between two chairs, one supporting the head and one the feet, and be so strong as to support people standing on the body. (Do not try this at home for yourself.)

The psychologist then persuaded his student to eat a raw onion after convincing him it was an apple. The student took two hefty bites from the onion and seemed to enjoy the taste—which is exactly the response one would expect from someone in good-quality hypnosis. At the end of the exercise, the student claimed to have been fully aware that he had, in fact, been eating an onion. It was only at this point that the tears formed in his eyes. There were no tears when he was "pretending."

The psychologist was saying, in effect, that the state of hypnosis does not exist, so why waste your time with it. He used terms like "social compliance" to explain away the ability of hypnotized subjects to display signs of having control of their own minds. He concluded by comparing hypnosis to the dodo bird and said that, like that ill-fated creature, hypnosis would, given time, fade away. We think not.

In any case, with something like hypnosis, what you call it is immaterial. It is what you do with it that is important. In our view, the skeptical psychologist's approach may or may not have been hypnotic, but the effects were clearly remarkable. If this were called hypnosis, it would be the same.

Transference in Hypnosis
Hypnotherapy has an advantage over psychoanalysis

With psychoanalysis, a patient can become dependent upon the therapist, either through the need to hand over responsibility to someone else or through transference, whereby the client "transfers" feelings for someone else onto the therapist. For instance, a client having, for example, angry feelings towards their mother, might unconsciously transfer the feelings to the therapist by placing the therapist in a mother role and then feeling rage towards the therapist.

This situation tends to crop up in longer term therapies and it can be a very powerful tool for enabling the client to get in touch with repressed emotions. In modern hypnotherapy, however, the short-term nature of the therapy and the focus on the client and away from the therapist, ensure that this transference and dependence does not occur. Within the parameters of this kit, the issue of transference does not even come up.

Change
Hypnosis empowers us to change ourselves, either with the help of others or on our own behalf

If there is one thing mankind is not keen on, it is change. Anyone who has ever studied the body's stress mechanism will know that all change elicits a stress response. The fact that you are reading this, indicates that you welcome change, at least on this occasion and on a level determined by you. One of the most efficient tools for enabling change to take place is hypnosis, and this has resulted in some harsh words on the subject from those who feel threatened.

Recently, a person of reasonably high profile launched a major assault against hypnotherapy because of the changes which took place in her husband after he had taken a course of hypnotherapy. It is alleged that these changes resulted in the husband leaving their relationship.

A certain bitterness on the part of the woman is understandable but, we feel, misdirected. All loving relationships are formed on a subconscious level. Relationship counsellors call it the "fit"; the general public often refers to it as "chemistry." Often, what attracts you to a partner is the subconscious recognition of a part of you that is missing. People who are complete opposites often form long-term, successful relationships.

As a relationship develops, and as the individuals themselves change, the fit also changes. If the individuals can accommodate these changes, the relationship is maintained. If only one partner changes—becomes more confident, develops intellectually or artistically, or whatever—and the other partner remains "stuck," tensions are set up within the relationship which may cause it to fail.

At times of stress within a relationship, it is natural for blame to be apportioned. Often affairs, lack of understanding, unreasonable behavior, or other factors may be cited as the reasons for the breakdown. In reality, each relationship is a deal, made on a subconscious level. Affairs are symptoms of the deal changing, not things that cause it to change. Although a great defence mechanism, blame within a relationship is inappropriate. So, blaming hypnotherapy for the break-up of a relationship is a bit like shooting the messenger for bringing bad news.

Control and Safety
Who is in control?

The word control invariably finds its way into the conversation whenever hypnosis is discussed and, in fact, control is basically what hypnosis is all about. But who is in control? In natural hypnosis (not drug-induced), at no time does the person in hypnosis give up control. Indeed, it is through hypnosis that the client learns how increasingly to take control of his or her own mind.

In the past, statements have been made about the ability to make a person in hypnosis do just about anything, regardless of their behavioral code. Despite evidence to the contrary, stories abound of assassins who have been programmed to carry out missions on behalf of others. Indeed, a great deal of money and time has been spent in attempts to get people to commit crimes while under someone else's control.

Religious cults are assumed to work in a similar manner, causing people to abandon lifelong beliefs and behave completely out of character. Rescuers of such people talk in terms of de-programming them.

Experts in the field are quite clear about the notion that it is possible to take control of someone's mind. While it can be shown that hypnosis could be used in this exploitive process, we emphasize that hypnosis alone does not work. Other requirements are more influential and involve factors like complete control of the subject's environment, the use of drugs depriving the subject of sleep for long periods, and working over a period of time to alter the subject's perception of reality. This leads to disorientation and, eventually, re-programming.

As you can see, this process falls well outside the scope of hypnosis and hypnotherapy. If complete mind control were possible merely by using hypnosis, hypnotists would have taken control of the world long before now!

Theatrical or stage hypnotists have a lot to answer for as they perpetuate the myth that it is possible to take control of someone's mind and force them into doing something against their will. What, in fact, occurs is that the stage hypnotist screens each of the volunteers in order to ascertain their ability to work with their imagination. Those most able and willing to go along with the outrageous suggestions propounded by the hypnotist are the ones the hypnotist will choose. If you have ever seen a live stage show, you will have noticed that out of a vast number of volunteers, the hypnotist will choose, say, ten or twelve, and out of these, only work with about four or five on individual routines. These are volunteers who enter into a contract of consent with the hypnotist: *they place themselves under hypnosis.*

Although each subject experiences the routine as a form of reality, they have agreed to let it happen.

What is more, would it not be a great excuse to be able to make a complete fool of yourself and then be able to blame someone or something else? If you have ever attended a party, you will have seen this sort of thinking in action, no hypnosis required, just a bit of alcohol perhaps. You might also suspect that at hypnotism shows or acts it is these same kinds of people who are called upon to perform the outrageous "hypnotic suggestions." This is, in fact, true and a stage hypnotist looks for tell-tale characteristics. It could be argued that a person who is prepared to behave in this way has the ability to "let go" without the need for the usual defences. On the other hand, it could be that the person wants to avoid reality. Either way, it makes for some interesting stage shows.

It is certainly true to say that a form of hypnosis can be used to assist in manipulation. Mass manipulation takes place twenty-four hours a day, uses a form of hypnosis, and is not only condoned by society but actively supported by it. It is not carried out by doctors, psychiatrists, psychologists, hypnotherapists, or any other kind of therapist. It is carried out by advertisers.

Mass Manipulation
Do advertisers and the media hypnotize us?

Many advertisements are designed to link a certain product with a positive feeling. The point is that, when you buy the product, you get the feeling—if you buy another brand, you do not. The feelings can range from "good" to "right" to "sexy," and all the positive feelings in between.

With television advertisements, the idea is that they should be viewed once or twice and then ignored. In this way, you take in the information on a conscious level, and then by "switching off" your conscious attention during further showings, you take in the information on a subconscious level—which is where your feelings come from. Some advertisers make their commercials so preposterous that you cannot bear to watch them more than once. From the advertiser's point of view, that is fine: you are still getting the message whether you like it or not.

Advertising has little to do with rational thought. On a thinking level, most commercials do not really work. For instance, advertisements for performance cars are usually aimed at the male section of the population. The message often goes something like this: if you drive this car, the super-deluxe-special-extra, it will enable you to drive through exotic places, enjoying admiring glances from the locals, and you will get the girl. In other words, you will enjoy the lifestyle you have always wished for.

Now, on a conscious, rational level, you realize that you probably cannot even afford such a car in the first place and, even if you could scrape the money together, it would probably adversely affect your humdrum lifestyle. If you could easily afford the car, you also know that ownership of such a car alone does not mean that you will get the girl. But, on a subconscious, emotional level, the concept feels kind of nice...

Over twenty years ago, there was a television commercial for a laxative which showed a woman enter a mobile library and ask for a book on biology because she was constipated! The idea was so staggeringly awful that the commercial itself was almost enough to induce mass diarrhea. Over twenty years have gone by since we last saw this commercial but the image (and the product) is vividly remembered. You might like to check this one out for yourself. The next time you are with a group of people, whistle a theme song or use a catch-phrase (they are not called catch-phrases for nothing) from a well-known product or program, and watch the reaction. At this point you will have, for a brief moment, influenced their minds in that you will have them thinking about something of your choosing without them wishing to do so. This simple example illustrates the extraordinary powers of suggestion.

A Recurring Theme
Why hypnotherapy is not encouraged in some quarters

An interesting but possibly sinister development has occured recently. Some states have legislated against the use of hypnosis except by doctors, psychiatrists and psychologists.

This throws up a number of extremely interesting issues which not everybody is willing to debate. Could it be that drug companies want to suppress the growth of hypnotherapy? Such companies pamper and support orthodox medicine because it is the doctors who issue and recommend their products. Hypnotherapists, on the other hand, may make the use of drugs redundant. This is not an irrational or cynical point of view. The large drug companies have a vested interest in limiting the number of practising hypnotherapists and they are certainly rich and powerful enough to exert political influence.

The current trend, particularly in the United States, of trying to prevent qualified hypnotherapists from practicing their skills, smacks of hypocrisy when we realize that responsible therapists help their clients to make positive changes within themselves by exercising more control over their own minds. It would seem that the government, media, and certain religious organizations quite freely use their own form of hypnosis in an attempt to manipulate those very same people. Of course, they would not dream of calling it hypnosis.

One school of thought is that when enough people begin to exercise control of their own lives and accept responsibility for their own health and well-being, when what scientists refer to as critical mass is reached, the system, which can only function by controlling those within it, will have to alter in a big way. There are too many vested interests, too much at stake, for the system to let this happen without fighting it every inch of the way. This scenario certainly seems to fit with what has been happening to hypnosis throughout the long and turbulent history of civilization.

Recent Developments

Changing consciousness is leading towards wider recognition of hypnosis

Nowadays, hypnosis is much more widely accepted, both by the medical profession and by the general public. Although, as you will have gathered, this acceptance has been a long time coming.

In the late 1980s a study was conducted by the Stanford Medical School into using hypnosis for pain relief. This was reported in *The New York Times*, stating that hypnosis could suppress the brain's perception of pain and that there was a sound basis for trying it in clinical use. The medical establishment has caught up at last! The medical profession has just discovered something that hypnotherapists have been doing for hundreds of years!

Hypnosis has also been acknowledged by other professions. Forensic hypnosis is used widely in some countries (particularly in America) by the police. This is now carefully monitored as it was soon realized that memories recalled in hypnosis can be imaginary or merely suggestions by the therapist.

Hypnosis is also widely used in sports to motivate people to excel—it has finally been acknowledged that any great golfer, tennis player, or individual athlete has an edge over an opponent when the mind is trained to play a positive role in their achievements

As the relevance and importance of hypnosis has become more widely acknowledged, various people have sought to preserve its good reputation and to prevent its misuse. In the last few years theatrical hypnosis has become extremely popular in Britain, although it is still banned in some countries. Because of misunderstanding by the general public in regard to the compliance of volunteers for these stage shows, and because of the misgivings that people have about the stage hypnotist taking control of their minds, these shows have given the profession of hypnotherapy a bad name. However, the main societies of stage hypnotists in Britain recently banded together to form a new organization in order to regulate the ethical use of stage hypnosis and to bring about better standards. It is true to say that we, although not altogether approving theatrical hypnosis, do actually know at least one American stage hypnotist, Ormond McGill, with whom we would trust our lives, whether in hypnosis or not.

At the present time, negotiations are taking place in Europe between umbrella organizations (such as the Institute of Complementary Medicine and the British Complementary Medicine Association) and government bodies to ensure that regulating procedures and training standards are agreed at some time in the future. When that happens, professional hypnotherapy will gain the credibility and esteem that it so richly deserves but which has eluded it throughout the last two centuries.

The Knock-on Effect
The multiple benefits of hypnosis

In the current climate of enthusiasm for holistic, drug-free therapies which complement conventional medicine, hypnotherapy is being used successfully to treat a wide range of problems. Many people are aware of the benefits of hypnotherapy in treating phobias, weight loss and smoking. But one of the aims of this book is to highlight areas of successful treatment which might not readily spring to mind when the word hypnotherapy is mentioned. For instance, are you aware that most physical problems can be quickly improved by using modern hypnotic techniques? This includes those physical problems which have a psychological element (which, in our experience, is most of them) and those which are purely physical—broken bones, torn ligaments and the like.

By better understanding how the subconscious mind works, we are able to direct the body's natural ability to heal itself to those areas which require the work. In speaking to clients over the years, it is amusing to note just how many believe that it is the hospital that fixes broken bones! It never seems to occur to them that the doctors just set the bones in place. It is in fact the subconscious which starts the growth process and, more importantly, switches it off again when the work is complete.

When speaking to clients about how the mind affects the body, they readily accept psychosomatic illness, but seem to have great difficulty in accepting psychosomatic wellness. Perhaps they are locked into a day-to-day routine where they are slaves to their mind rather than realizing that the mind is there to serve them. It seems a shame that most people go through life never having known that this is the case and, as a result, never having learned how to take control.

This lack of understanding means that many clients come to us for hypnotherapy for out-of-the-ordinary complaints only when they have reached a state of absolute desperation. Alternatively, having come with a more mundane problem, the hypnotherapist often indicates that other problems might be dealt with during the course of therapy.

One of the more interesting of such cases concerned a client who presented himself to us with an arthritic hip. During the initial consultation, it transpired that he was also dyslexic. Mike, a forty-six-year-old martial arts master, had developed some excellent coping skills over the years to overcome the difficulty he had with reading. The one thing he had great trouble with, however, was his inability to deal with numbers. Telephone numbers were a real problem. As he could only manage three digits at a time, and had to spend a considerable amount of time memorizing each set of three, he found that by the time he was ready to dial the second set of digits, the telephone would often have switched off. He told us that on one occasion he attempted to dial a nearby town only to end up talking to someone in New Zealand! Good news for the telephone company but bad news for Mike!

When it was mentioned that perhaps we could do some work with the dyslexia during a session when we were working on the hip, the look Mike gave suggested that he thought it was us who needed the therapy. The work with the dyslexia took some ten minutes, at the end of which we wrote down a telephone number and asked him to go into reception and dial it. This he duly did and he has been dialing numbers and reading books with no problem ever since. And his hip is doing nicely, too!

Such is the power of the mind. When Mike learned how to start taking control of his, it completely changed his life. And the good news is that Mike is by no means an isolated case. This sort of work goes on, quietly in the background, day in and day out. Although conventional medicine is reluctant to acknowledge the sheer scale of the changes which are being effected with hypnosis, the results cannot be denied.

The Views of Eminent Hypnotherapists
Positive words to allay fears and doubts

The benefits of hypnotherapy are only too obvious to us but you may still have some lingering doubts before moving on through the book. Here are some reassuring words from experts.

"As to self-hypnosis, many thousands have learned it, I have yet to hear a report of any bad results from its use."

Leslie LeCron,
psychologist and authority on hypnosis.

"Platinov, an associate of Pavlov, who used hypnosis for over fifty years, in more than fifty thousand cases, reported: 'We have never observed any harmful influence on the patient which could be ascribed to the methods of hypnotherapy, or any tendency towards the development of unstable personality traits, weakening of the will, or pathological urge for hypnosis.'"

Dr. William S. Kroger,
author of *Clinical & Experimental Hypnosis*.

"The so-called dangers from hypnosis are imaginary. Although I have hypnotised many hundreds of patients, I

have never seen any ill effects from its use."

Dr. Julius Grinker

"Hypnotism is absolutely safe. There is no known case on record of harmful results from its therapeutic use."

Rafael Rhodes,
psychologist and author of *Therapy Through Hypnosis.*

"In over thirty-seven years of practice, and ten years of teaching hypnotherapy, I have come to the conclusion that fear of hypnosis is generated by those who have no intrinsic understanding of what hypnosis is, nor an open mind to allow them to explore this wonderful human gift for the benefit of mankind."

Bill Atkinson-Ball,
founder of The Atkinson-Ball College of
Hypnotherapy and HypnoHealing.

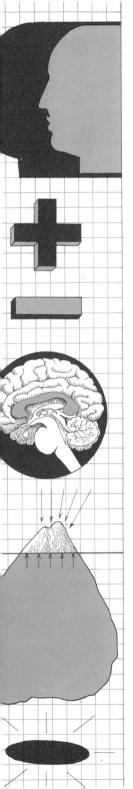

Chapter Three

Know Your Own Mind

Few things are as fascinating as what goes on inside our heads. The physical structure of the brain is immensely complex and the many functions of this pallid, spongy organ are truly amazing. You may find some of the following information on what makes you tick both revealing and exciting.

The brain itself is similar to a computer. It weighs about 3 pounds (1.4 kilograms) and contains in the region of 30 billion neurons. Neurons are like the circuits in a computer and each one is a collection of molecules which act together to process information. The sheer number of neurons in the brain gives you some idea of the potential of brain/mind power. Interestingly, new ideas in biochemistry on the mind/body connection suggest that, as all the organs of the body produce the same chemicals as the brain when it is thinking, then it is logical to assume that the whole body combined makes up the mind and that it is not just confined to the brain.

These theories are not universally accepted, however, and from the viewpoint of neuro-surgeons, without the brain there would be no mind. Research by neurologists and neuro-surgeons indicates that the subconscious mind is located in three specific areas of the brain. These are as follows:

• The temporal lobe of the cerebral cortex, located near the temple. This houses the memory as has been proven by surgeons who have released various memories by stimulating nerve cells in the area. Stimulation of different nerve cells results in the recall of different memories.

• The cerebellum, located at the back of the brain stem. This houses the co-ordinating, blending and detailing functions of the voluntary muscles, that is, those muscles used in learning to crawl, walk, tying

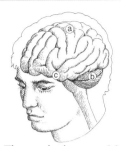

The cerebral cortex (a), cerebellum (b), and hypothalamus (c) of the human brain.

The Functions of the Subconscious Mind

How hypnosis can influence the workings of the subconscious mind

laces and so on. Neurologists have found that when the cerebellum has been injured, these movements become jerky and uncoordinated.

• The hypothalamus, located deep in the brain, just above the pituitary gland. This controls the major part of the subconscious mind. It is the integrating centre for the autonomic nervous system which regulates the glands and all involuntary activities. The hypothalamus directs a great deal of subconscious activity because it is triggered by emotion.

It is often said that each of us uses only a small percentage of our mind—Einstein estimated that we work with no more than ten per cent of it. No wonder then, that the mind has been referred to as the "mental iceberg" as so much of its activity is below the surface and so much of its capacity is unused. One role the subconscious mind plays is to act as our servant as far as habits are concerned. We learn at an early age to walk, to eat our food with a knife and fork, to ride a bike, and so on. These habit patterns are never forgotten. We just do them automatically. But what are the less obvious jobs of the subconscious mind and how can hypnosis help?

• The subconscious mind controls all the involuntary functions of the body such as digestion, breathing, heart rate, temperature and so on. This is obviously all done without any conscious thought. It is widely accepted now that anxiety, stress and tension can negatively affect these functions, and these bad effects are known as psychosomatic illnesses. It stands to reason therefore that, as hypnosis can directly contact the subconscious mind, then hypnosis can bring about recovery.

• The subconscious mind can be regarded as our own personal computer, our memory bank. It stores every-

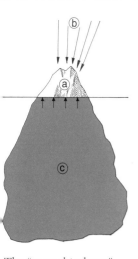

The "mental iceberg:"
The conscious mind (a)
which receives external
stimuli (b), occupies
only a small part of the
brain. The subconscious
mind (c) occupies the
bulk of the brain and
records past experiences.

The Power of the Subconscious
How thoughts dominate our actions

thing that we have seen, heard, done and experienced. Nothing is ever erased unless the brain is injured in some way. Through hypnosis, memories can be retrieved, but, a word of warning: do not forget that some memories have been "hidden" or buried by the subconscious for our own protection.

• All our emotions are contained within the subconscious mind, and one of the rules of the mind is that emotion is usually stronger than reason. It would seem therefore that we are at the mercy of our subconscious mind, that is until we learn to take control of it through hypnosis.

• The subconscious mind contains our ability to use our imagination. When you think about it, worry is only negative imagination. Through hypnosis, one's imagination can be utilized to think of how good things could be rather than how bad they could be.

• Our subconscious mind provides us with motivation; it directs the physical and emotional energy which we fuel by eating. For instance, if you decide to give up smoking, your conscious mind is responsible for this goal selection. Unless the subconscious mind releases the energy to make this happen, you will probably either start smoking again or use a displacement activity such as eating or drinking. With the help of hypnosis, the subconscious mind can direct energy in a positive way to help us to fulfil our goals.

Whatever action we take is first of all determined by our thoughts so, if we change our thoughts, we can change the way we behave. The subconscious mind does not like changes but in hypnosis it can be persuaded to make them once it realizes that they are beneficial.

The strength of the mind has been demonstrated in a highly effective way by Anthony Robbins who runs seminars all over the world on what he calls "personal power." As a simple illustration to prove the power of the mind, seminar participants have been able to walk over red hot coals without burning their feet. Most people would say that this is physically impossible but with the power of the mind, nothing is impossible.

As Napoleon Hill, who wrote the book *Think and Grow Rich*, said, "Whatever the mind can conceive, and believe, it can achieve," and it is true to say that most of the people who succeed in life are those who know the power of their own mind. Those who fail are the ones who spend most of their lives searching outside, expecting help from other people, rather than looking at themselves.

Once we can communicate with our subconscious mind—through hypnosis—then we can begin to realize that all the answers are there within ourselves. The concept that all the faculties we need are already within us is a powerful one to press home.

Whatever you want in life, it is important to know what it is and to have a goal. Thoughts have a boomerang effect. If we think negative thoughts, then we attract negative things happening to us. Likewise, if we visualize good things, then we attract the positive. The more powerful and intense a thought is, then the more powerful and intense the outcome will be.

Imagination

How images change the way we think and behave

Imagination is one of the most powerful mental abilities that we possess as human beings and it can be both positive and negative.

Imagination relates to our beliefs about ourselves, based on our past experience. When we feel "stuck" or cannot "see" our way out of a situation, then the full force of our imagination comes into effect with words like "what if" and "if only." What we do is map out our own future in a very negative way, programming ourselves for future problems, unhappiness and general feelings of being unfulfilled. In hypnosis, it is possible to open the corridor to new ways of positive thinking.

If we can discipline our minds to imagine in a positive way, then we are able to empower ourselves to achieve what we want. How many times do we say to ourselves "I just can't see myself being able to do that." If, however, we can visualize ourselves doing exactly what we want, then we are half way to reaching the goal.

It is well known amongst psychologists and hypnotherapists that imagination is far more powerful than reason. This is hardly surprising since imagination comes from the subconscious, the largest part of the mind, whereas reason comes from the smaller, conscious part. When we can take control of our own subconscious mind, with the use of positive imagination, then the possibility of success becomes assured.

Through imagination we have the power to choose. Maybe we could use the analogy of electricity: the use of electricity can either warm us up or it can electrocute us. Likewise, our imagination can enhance our lives or it can blight us. In hypnosis, the conscious mind, which is so often the negative stumbling block, can be by-passed and the subconscious can be accessed to provide a more positive imagination. Hypnosis can literally change our "frame of mind." How much more refreshing it is to say, "I can and I will" rather than "I can't."

Inner Dialogue
The powers and effects of words

The subconscious mind is surprisingly literal, For example, if we constantly think of someone as "a pain in the neck" then there is a good chance that this statement will manifest itself physically. Likewise, such phrases as "I am sick to my stomach" and, "He's getting on my nerves" can also have similar adverse effects on the body if they are allowed to become part of one's inner dialogue for any length of time. They actually become a subconscious belief.

This may sound ridiculous but let us give you an

example. A client arrived on our doorstep with her head turned completely to one side. Her problem was spasmodic torticollis (commonly known as wry neck) In hypnosis it was found out that her husband had had an affair and the phrase that had been going through her head was, "I just can't face up to this."

Perhaps an even more dramatic example was a well reported case in America of a young lady who had gone into a coma and had remained in it for several years. The story hit the headlines because her parents wanted to turn off the life-support machine, and there was a great deal of controversy about whether this should be done. However, when her diary was examined, the entry for the day before she went into the coma read, "I wish I could go to sleep and never wake up."

So, we obviously have to be very careful about the way we think and we cannot stress too much just how powerful an effect these kinds of negative phrases can have on a person's health and well-being. It is vitally important that we recognize the need to control our own inner dialogue and also to acknowledge that the connection between mind and body is inseparable.

Emile Coué, the eminent French psychologist, recognized this as far back as the early part of the century. He encouraged all his patients to repeat at least six times every day, "Every day in every way I am getting better and better."

If we continually give positive statements to our subconscious mind (even though our conscious mind may not accept them to start off with) then sooner or later it will act upon them. Repetition is how we learned numerous things as a child and there is no reason why that should change in adulthood.

It is, however, extremely difficult to start thinking in a positive way when perhaps for the whole of our lives we have been conditioned to think in a negative way. This is where hypnosis can play an important role because the subconscious mind can be contacted directly and reprogrammed without negative interference from the conscious.

Merely understanding the workings of the mind, and the power of inner dialogue, can bring about immediate enlightenment to most people. It can even become a stepping stone for bringing about a return to physical well-being. After all, we believe that over ninety per cent of illnesses are psychosomatic.

Mind Over Matter
The placebo effect

It has been estimated that at least thirty per cent of patients respond positively to placebos. This occurs not just in pain relief but also with conditions such as heart disease and cancer. When a placebo is effective, a person genuinely believes that they are going to get better and the body responds by manufacturing the necessary chemicals to relieve the condition.

Placebos were occasionally used in the First World War when supplies of morphine ran out and injured soldiers were injected with water. They were told that this was a new drug that was ten times stronger than morphine. The result was that many soldiers felt no pain at all.

A few years ago, the British Medical Research Council did a trial to see if placebos could prevent high blood pressure. One lady in the trial was given a placebo which she took for five years. During that time her blood pressure went down and remained at a safe level. At the end of the trial, she stopped taking the placebo and her blood pressure went up. The strange twist at the end of the tale is that the doctors then gave her a drug for high blood pressure! Why didn't they put her back on the placebo?

Even the color of placebos are important. A report in the *British Medical Journal* stated that red placebos were better for pain relief than any other color!

The placebo effect illustrates very well the effect the mind can have on the body and how the subconscious mind can produce its own natural healing energies.

In recent years, surgeons have begun to realize that patients having surgery under general anesthesia are subconciously wide open to anything that is said in their presence. If positive suggestions are made while a patient is having surgery, doctors have learned that there are likely to be fewer post-operative complications, and less need for painkilling drugs.

Now that you have an idea of the power of your mind, you may begin to understand why you do some of the things you do. This basic knowledge will better enable you to take the next steps in your exploration of hypnosis.

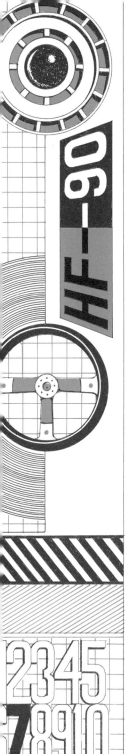

Chapter Four

First Practical Steps

You are now ready to embark on a journey of discovery, self-improvement and even enlightenment. You have come a long way—to reach this stage, you have already shown not only an interest in hypnosis, but also a willingness to experiment. It is this willingness that will make your hypnosis more likely to succeed. You are now almost ready to use the tape that comes with this book.

There is one fact that we would like to reiterate at this point: you cannot be hypnotized against your will. Let us once again remind you of your control while in hypnosis, using the analogy of the driverless car (see Introduction).

- YOU switch on the ignition—equivalent to making contact with your sub-conscious mind.
- YOU steer the car—equivalent to giving suggestions to your subconscious mind.
- YOU can then accelerate—equivalent to programming your subconscious mind for personal growth.
- Or YOU can brake—equivalent to bringing yourself out of hypnosis.
- Whatever you choose, YOU are the driver—equivalent to you being in control of your subconscious mind.

Put your conscious mind at ease before you play the tape by running through the following points.

- You have been in hypnosis many times before. You may not have recognized it as hypnosis—maybe you thought of it as a daydream, a reverie, a meditation, but it was in fact hypnosis. In other words, any time that you are doing something that you are not consciously thinking about, you are in a form of hypnosis.

• There is no way that you are going to get "stuck" in hypnosis while listening to the tape—you can awaken yourself at any time if you so desire. For instance, if the telephone rings, or someone talks to you, you will be fully aware of the situation and can open your eyes and be wide awake, instantly.

• The tape has been specifically designed for optimum effect. Side A is a traditional induction; Side B is a different kind of induction that is designed to reinforce the effect of Side A. Although Side B offers you an alternative means of going into hypnosis, it is important that you listen to Side A first or else it will make little sense. Once you are familiar with both sides, you can choose which side you listen to the most. Both sides of the tape are designed to hold the attention of the subconscious mind for about twenty-five minutes. After years of research, the authors consider this an ideal time span for hypnosis.

• Most important of all: never forget that you are the one who is in control. At no time do you give up your free will, become unconscious or lose your memory.

Dos and Don'ts

• DO sit down in a comfortable chair and let yourself relax with the tape.
• DO set aside time each day to play the tape on a regular basis. Twice a day is ideal.
• DO enjoy the tape by just letting the process unfold rather than trying to make anything happen.
• **DO NOT play the tape while driving, operating machinery or doing anything which requires your attention or motor skills.**
• DO NOT worry if you fall asleep or if your mind wanders while listening to the tape. If you cannot remember what was on the tape after listening to it, that is okay—your subconscious mind will still have absorbed the beneficial suggestions and will be able to act upon them.

How You Can Expect to Feel

• If you have never listened to a hypnosis tape before, you may find that you feel wary, skeptical, fearful, or just plain curious before you switch it on.

• While listening to the tape you may feel pleasantly relaxed, lethargic, or, again, just curious.

• After you have listened to the tape you should feel totally relaxed and relieved that at last you have found something that you know can help you.

Preparation
The importance of comfort

All you have to do is to find yourself a comfortable chair or, if you prefer, you can lie down on a bed. The "correct" position is the one in which you feel the most comfortable. Then, just adopt an attitude of mind that you are going to allow yourself twenty minutes or so of peace and quiet.

Let us stress that there is no need for a darkened room, for a specific temperature, for you to be covered with a blanket, or for music to be playing in the background. In other words, you do not need any special effects.

The Hypnotic Induction
The instructions on Side A of the tape

The following outline provides an idea of the structure of the induction on Side A of the tape that accompanies this book and the purpose of each step. The tape contains more explicit spoken instructions for you to follow, taking you carefully through each stage of the process in a soothing, relaxing voice that will enable you to experience good quality hypnosis. Once you are familiar with what is on the tape, you can move on to putting yourself into hypnosis unaided (Chapter Five), and ultimately you can learn to address specific problems (Chapter Six).

Step 1
Physical Relaxation

The first two or three minutes of Side A concern physical relaxation. First, you are asked to close your eyes in order to aid your concentration, then you are encouraged to tense and relax individual groups of muscles,

starting with the feet and working up to the scalp.
PURPOSE: Mind and body are related—when one is relaxed, it is easier for the other to relax as well. This exercise also makes you aware of where you have been holding tension in specific parts of your body.

Step 2
Eye Closure

This part of the induction asks you to fix your eyes on a spot on the ceiling, looking up as far as you can without lifting your head. While you are doing this, you are asked to start counting backwards from five hundred. Count to yourself silently and rhythmically and, if you lose count, just pick it up at any number—you will not be counting for long.
PURPOSE: This is a way of tiring your eyes, allowing them to close in their own time. The procedure occupies your conscious mind while allowing easier access to your subconscious mind.

Step 3
Counting Down

At this stage, numbers are counted for you from one to ten. As each number is mentioned, you can let yourself enjoy a deeper feeling of both mental and physical relaxation.
PURPOSE: This is an effective way of improving the quality of your hypnosis. The key to this section is your willingness to let it happen, which then prepares you for the next step. The more you play the tape, the more you practice the technique, the better the end result.

Step 4
Using Your Imagination

In this part of the tape, a garden will be described in general terms and you will be asked to imagine how it looks. There is no right way or wrong way to do this exercise; however you "see," "sense," or just pretend that you are in a garden, is fine.
PURPOSE: This sequence allows your natural creative ability—that is your subconscious mind—to come to the fore, enabling you to enjoy the sensations of being in a lovely setting, and experiencing an inner sense of peace and tranquillity.

Step 5
Suggestions

As you continue to enjoy these lovely feelings of peace and comfort, you are now in a position to direct positive suggestions to your receptive subconscious mind. You are asked to picture yourself looking confident, fit and healthy.

PURPOSE: By framing these suggestions, your subconscious mind readily accepts and acts upon them, enabling positive changes to take place within you.

Step 6
The Post-Hypnotic Suggestion

At the end of the tape you are given a suggestion that when you want to take yourself into self-hypnosis, all you have to do is to turn your eyes up to a spot high on the ceiling, count from one to ten, take a long deep breath and as you breathe out allow your eyes to close right down and say to yourself the words "HYPNOSIS NOW." That is all you have to do. You will find yourself once again on your garden bench, enjoying the relaxation, being aware of the garden and everything in it.

PURPOSE: The post-hypnotic suggestion helps you to achieve hypnosis within seconds, to improve the quality of it and of course to be able to go into hypnosis all by yourself—in other words, you will be able to practice self-hypnosis.

Step 7
The Wake-up

This topic may engender one of your greatest fears regarding hypnosis. "Will I ever wake up again?" As you listen to the tape, you have no fear of this since the voice on the tape guides you by counting backwards from ten to one and telling you that at one you will be wide awake and fully alert. When you are in self-hypnosis, you do exactly the same thing for yourself, remembering to tell yourself that you are wide awake and alert, feeling rested and refreshed, and any other positive statement that is appropriate.

PURPOSE: This gently brings you out of hypnosis while ensuring that all the positive benefits of the hypnosis remain with you. As we have said before, if an emergency arose while you were in hypnosis then you would automatically wake up.

Side B of the tape is not so much a formal hypnotic induction but more an exercise in awareness. It reinforces Side A but can be used as an alternative to induce hypnosis.

• The first section exercises your mind by focusing your concentration on different parts of your body (as opposed to relaxing them as is suggested in Side A). This focused concentration automatically enables you to enter into an altered state of consciousness which is in fact hypnosis.

• The second section allows you to take your mind outside itself, as it were, to look at yourself and your surroundings from a different perspective. This is an important starting point along your pathway to personal development as it enables you to look at yourself and any problems you may have more objectively.

• The third section contains specific affirmations for greater confidence, something that most people need in one aspect or another.

• The fourth section is a repeat of the post-hypnotic suggestion on Side A. This enables you to take yourself into hypnosis in the future.

The whole purpose of the tape is to help you within a very short space of time to enter into hypnosis for yourself, by yourself. At that stage you are truly independent and will not need to play the tape regularly.

Now, p-l-a-y t-h-e t-a-p-e! We suggest that you play both sides at least two or three times before you use the post-hypnotic suggestion, so that you can acquaint yourself fully with the experience of being in hypnosis.

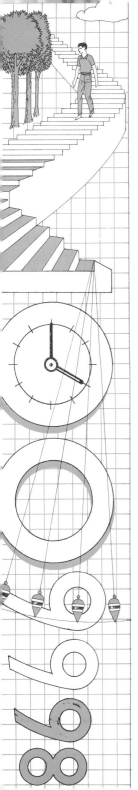

Chapter Five

Using the Post-Hypnotic Suggestion

Now comes the testing time: you are about to go into hypnosis all by yourself. Remember that the instructions you have received on the tape are now firmly implanted in your subconscious mind.

Here is the procedure.

• Sit yourself down in a comfortable chair, at a time when you know that you are not going to be disturbed.

• Take a few moments to make yourself physically comfortable in the chair.

• Turn your eyes up to a spot high on the ceiling.

• Count from one to ten, take a long deep breath, and as you breathe out allow your eyelids to close right down and say to yourself the words *"HYPNOSIS NOW."*

• Now find yourself once again sitting on your bench in your own private garden. Be aware of the trees and shrubs surrounding the garden and see the sunlight glinting on the water in the ornamental pond. Be aware of the flowers, the grass and the feelings of comfort and relaxation you have each time you come into this garden.

• When you are ready, awaken yourself in the same way that we do on the tape—by counting backwards from ten to one and telling yourself on the count of one that you are wide awake and alert.

That is all there is to it.

Now there is a chance that at this point you may very well say to yourself that the quality of hypnosis was not as good as when you were listening to the tape. But remember that learning self-hypnosis is like learning any other new skill: the more you do it, the better it gets. So, we urge you to practice your self-hypnosis on a regular basis, preferably once or twice a day. In a very short space of time, you will amaze yourself at how proficient you are.

Just in case we have not got our message across, let us return to the analogy of the car.

• You have just acquired a brand new car—equivalent to the new skill you have of self-hypnosis.

• After a considerable length of time you decide to start up the car but you have left it so long that the battery has gone dead—equivalent to your trying to do self-hypnosis weeks or months after you first played the tape.

• You have a change of heart and decide to recharge the battery, taking the car out for a run every day to keep all its mechanical parts running smoothly—equivalent to practicing self-hypnosis every day.

Setting a Time Limit
The subconscious is aware of time

"What if I fall asleep? What if I can't wake up?" These may be questions that you have asked yourself. Do not worry—the worst that can happen is that you fall asleep if you are tired. In which case, you would simply wake up as usual from ordinary sleep. But what if you only have a certain amount of time to spare to go into hypnosis? The answer is to set yourself a specific time limit to be in hypnosis—your subconscious mind is very aware of time and you can easily program it to wake yourself up on cue.

As you enter hypnosis and say *"HYPNOSIS NOW"* to yourself, add the words *"for ten minutes"* or for whatever time limit you want to set for yourself.

You will not need to awaken yourself consciously this time by counting backwards from ten to one—your subconscious mind will automatically do that for you. You will astonish yourself at how easy and effective this is. Do not take our word for it—try it for yourself and be amazed!

After you have practiced self-hypnosis a few times, you may be asking yourself how you can take yourself to a deeper level, remembering that the more relaxed you are, the easier it becomes to work with your subconscious mind.

Deepening Techniques
The deeper the hypnosis, the more relaxed you become

Here are a few suggestions for you to try out once you have established yourself on your garden bench.

• Just raise your right arm a few inches up into the air and as you drop it heavily back into your lap, give yourself the suggestion that you will take yourself three times deeper. Just decide to let it happen.

• Open your eyes and as you close them again, give yourself the suggestion that you will take yourself three times deeper.

• Take a long deep breath and as you breathe out, give yourself the suggestion that you will take yourself three times deeper.

• Just say to yourself the word *"deeper"* two or three times, telling yourself that you will take yourself deeper each time you say the word.

• Sitting on your garden bench, do some counting. This time, count from one hundred backwards and after you say each number to yourself, add the words *"deeper and deeper."* Look up into the sky above the trees surrounding your garden and imagine that you can see numbers side by side ranging from one hundred downwards. As soon as you start counting the numbers, notice that each one gets smaller and fainter than the one before. By the time you get to ninety five or ninety four, the numbers just disappear. This level of hypnosis is called somnambulism because when it was first observed the hypnotic subject gave off signs very similar to a somnambule (a sleepwalker) We know now that it is nothing like sleepwalking but the name has stuck.

These suggestions are among the simplest and quickest ways of deepening hypnosis but you may care to use some visualization techniques to achieve the same effect.

• Imagine that you are watching a pendulum swinging to and fro. Slow down the rhythm of the pendulum to relax even further and tell yourself that you are going deeper all the time you are watching that pendulum.

• As you sit on your garden bench, imagine that you are watching a fluffy white cloud in the sky and that it forms itself into the semblance of the word *"sleep."* Let it drift away on the breeze and then replace it with another cloud which again forms the word *"sleep."* Carry on in this way until you have reached the depth of hypnosis at which you feel comfortable.

• Imagine that you are walking slowly down a very long staircase and tell yourself that each step you take takes you deeper into hypnosis.

• Imagine that you are entering an elevator at the top of a very tall building. Go down in the elevator and watch the indicator as you pass each floor. With each number that comes up, go deeper into hypnosis. Obviously, do not use this visualization if you have a fear of lifts or enclosed spaces (see Chapter Seven for information on how phobias can be treated).

You may like to experiment with some visualizations of your own to deepen your hypnosis. Just find something that seems right and comfortable to you.

Measuring the Depth of your Hypnosis
How to use a ruler

As in all our techniques, simplicity is of the essence and nothing could be simpler than this next exercise. It stands to reason that if you are going to measure something, then you need a ruler. You need to tell yourself in hypnosis that a ruler will appear standing vertically in front you, numbered from zero at the top to one hundred at the bottom. The nearer you are to one hundred the deeper you are into hypnosis.

• After you have taken yourself down to your garden bench, count from one to three and tell yourself that on the count of three you can see a ruler standing upright in front of you.

• Again, count to yourself from one to three and tell yourself that on the count of three a number will stand out on the ruler equivalent to the quality of your relaxation.

• You can now deepen your hypnosis, using one of the deepening techniques already mentioned. You can either raise a hand and let it fall, open your eyes and then close them, or take a long deep breath. Tell yourself each time as you make one of those physical movements that you will double your relaxation.

• After each physical movement, count from one to three and check the measurement on your ruler. You can take yourself further and further down that ruler to the level at which you feel comfortable, or indeed to your optimum level of one hundred.

• When you have reached your desired level, suggest to yourself that the next time you take yourself into hypnosis you will go directly to that level.

• Lastly, remember to put your ruler away for safe keeping so that you can use it again on subsequent occasions.

By using this simple method of measurement you will quickly realize that you are genuinely taking control of your own hypnosis—you can now gauge its depth and deepen it as and when required.

Making Affirmations
The power of talking to yourself

As we have mentioned before, what we are and how we react to events and to other people is all dictated by earlier programming. Some of that programming has perhaps left undesirable results or, possibly, you may just want to reinforce some of the positive traits you already have. In any event, the chances are that you are keen to start putting new programs into your subconscious mind. The first way we can look at programming is through affirmation or talking to ourselves.

We all talk to ourselves a lot of the time and this inner dialogue is powerful stuff—so powerful that it can affect everything that we say or do.

As an example, let us suppose that you lack confidence in one or more areas of your life. You probably say to yourself negative statements like, *"I'll never be any good at that."* The more you say such things, the more you actually believe that you are useless. With the use of hypnosis, however, this sort of vicious circle can be broken.

If, while in hypnosis, you repeat the simple affirmation, *"I am confident,"* you can change the way you think about yourself. It sounds simple and it is, but remember that in hypnosis you talk directly to your subconscious mind and, if you repeat the affirmation time and time again, every part of your mind will eventually believe it.

We devote a whole section to confidence in Chapter Six but we hope that you're getting the message now as to how you can talk yourself into doing (or not doing) anything.

Hopefully, you have some ideas yourself of the kind of programming you would like to do and the affirmations that you need. There are, however, a few rules that need to be observed before you begin using an affirmation

• Keep the affirmation in the present. It is important that whatever statement you make is in the present tense. That is, you affirm it as though you have already achieved it so that the subconscious knows that this is something to be acted upon immediately. Do not use the future tense, i.e., *"I will be..."*

• Keep motivated. It is equally important that you convince the subconscious mind that the required change will produce a positive benefit, so tell it why. For example, you might say, *"I am becoming a non-smoker because I wish to be healthy, I wish to be in control and I wish to be free."*

• Keep it simple. The subconscious mind is like a child and it cannot comprehend long intellectual phrases. Therefore, keep your language simple but exciting. For example, *"I feel good, I feel great, I am happy."*

• Keep it positive. We have talked already of how so much of our earlier programming is negative, so the last thing you want to do is to put into your programming any phrases that hint at the negative such as, *"My headache disappears when I wake up."* Far better to say, *"As I relax more, my head becomes clearer."*

• Keep on repeating. The subconscious mind needs to be reminded again and again of what it should be doing. But do not fall into the trap of using the same words all the time. Use synonyms: *"I am becoming slim, I am gaining a slender figure."*

• Keep it specific. Tell your subconscious mind exactly what you want. If you want to lose weight, then let your subconscious mind know exactly what weight and size you want to be.

• Keep it to one thing at a time. Maybe you have many areas in which you wish to make changes but do not try to do everything at once. Start with the one that is most easy, change that first and then move on to others. If you make a suggestion that you are becoming more confident, then that will obviously help in all aspects of your future changes. If, on the other hand, you feel that you already have plenty of confidence and just want to work on becoming a non-smoker, then stick with that.

• Keep it realistic. Remember that confidence without competence can be a dangerous thing. It would be wrong to suggest that you could be a world skiing champion if you have never been on the slopes before. However, if you already have expertise in a particular sport or activity, then a suitable affirmation would be, *"As I grow in confidence, and as I relax more, then I become a better tennis player,"* or whatever.

Visualization
Seeing yourself differently

The second way we can look at programming is through visualization. We often say things to ourselves like, *"I just couldn't see myself doing that."* Maybe if we could see ourselves doing desired activities, then that might substitute the starting block for the stumbling block.

In hypnosis, you have direct access to your subconscious mind of which a part is your imagination. It figures that using your imagination in hypnosis can be very powerful and it is more than just possible to use it in a positive way.

Let us suppose, for instance, that you are quite a bit overweight. You undoubtedly see yourself as being fat every time you look in the mirror. You perceive that you are fat when you think about yourself and however much you want to lose weight, however many diets you go on, however much you deprive yourself of food, you still know that you are fat. That picture of yourself is well embedded into your mind. But just suppose that from now on, every time you take yourself into hypnosis you give your subconscious mind a picture of the way you want to be, maybe even a picture of how you used to be when you were slim, then don't you think that your subconscious mind might soon get the message and start having different ideas as to the real you, the inner you, the slim you that is inside you? That is just an example of how a positive picture can be used to change your inner concept of yourself.

Guided Fantasies
How to expand your imagination

A wonderful way of by-passing the conscious mind, of taking yourself deeper into hypnosis, of accessing your subconscious mind and achieving a therapeutic outcome, is to use guided fantasies. The following two fantasies are written out for you verbatim—all you have to do is read a passage to yourself a couple of times and then take yourself into hypnosis and let your mind do the rest. Alternatively, you could read it out aloud onto a tape and then play it back to yourself when you are in hypnosis. Only use one fantasy at a time.

Imagine that you are standing on a grassy knoll overlooking the sea. It is early morning and the sun is just rising over the horizon.

In front of you is a path leading down to a beach. Start walking down the path, slowly and carefully, feeling the sand and the pebbles beneath your feet. Breathe in the fresh sea air, relaxing more and more as you meander down the path. As you get nearer to the beach, hear the waves lapping gently on the sand and listen to the screech of the gulls as they circle overhead.

Now you are on the beach itself, in your own private world, in harmony with your surroundings and at peace with yourself. Walk along the beach, looking at your footprints in the virgin sand, until you come to a sheltered place in the dunes. Sink down into the soft warm sand, facing outwards towards the sea. Feel the fine soft sand as you let it trickle between your fingers. Be aware of the sun gently caressing your body and let the warm, healing rays soothe and relax you.

As you gaze ahead towards the horizon, you notice a flock of gulls soaring and swooping above the waves. You watch them for a while admiring their white plumage and their freedom. You wonder what it would be like to be one of them.

Imagine that you are looking at yourself, resting there in the sand. See yourself warm and protected by the sand dunes. Then rise up. Rise even higher and just drift gently and naturally towards the flock of gulls feeling as you drift upwards and nearer towards them the strength and the power of your wings. Most of all, relish the freedom that your wings give you.

Find that pure joy of knowing that you, too, can soar higher and higher, above the clouds towards the sun. Then slowly swoop down towards the sea until you feel your feet gently skimming the water, before once more you soar upwards again, realizing that you have the ability to fly wherever you want to go. Feel the power within you, knowing that there are no limits up here in the blue sky.

As you look inland towards the shore, you see on a solitary rock the outline of the Great White Gull, the wisest and most powerful bird of all. He has watched you grow, watched you in your quest for perfection, and he knows you better than you know yourself. He is the one who can answer any question you care to put to him.

Fly towards him, formulating a question in your mind as you go. As you come to rest on the rock beside him you know that here you can gain the knowledge that you need. Ask your question and wait for his answer.

When you are sure that you have all the answers you need, just slowly and peacefully drift back towards the sand dunes, shedding the feel of those wings until you arrive at at a point where you can see yourself sitting there in the sand. Now place yourself immediately above your image and slip gently back inside yourself, taking with you those memories of achievement, of freedom, and the knowledge that you have gained.

The purpose of the passage is fourfold.

• To increase your relaxation when in hypnosis.

• To expand your awareness and thereby your imagination.

• To give your subconscious mind an idea of freedom and to convince it of your ability to achieve what you want in a symbolic way.

• To enable you to ask a question of the Great White Gull (in other words, your own subconscious mind).

The next guided fantasy could be described as an exercise for spring-cleaning the attics of your mind. It is designed to get rid of negative thoughts, feelings and emotions, and to replace them with positive ones.

Imagine that you are sitting on a warm sunny beach. It is the sort of day when everyone seems to be at peace with the world. Other people on the beach are playing or splashing in the water and you are just watching them quietly. You are wondering why you are not feeling as happy as everyone else seems to be.

You somehow know that you have feelings and thoughts inside your head that are stopping you from enjoying this perfect summer's day. Some of these thoughts may be in connection with past events or they may be to do with what is happening in your life right now. Whatever the feelings are, you know they are negative.

You notice that to one side of you, lying there in the sand, there are several pebbles. Some of these are small but others are quite large and as you look at them, you realize that they represent some of the negative thoughts within you. They might represent just general negative feelings or they could represent something more specific like anger, frustration, resentment, low self-esteem, guilt, lack of confidence, self-punishment, or anything else that springs to your mind.

You pick up the first pebble, being fully aware of what negative aspect of you that it represents, and decide that you really do not need it any more. There is only one thing to do, and that is to get rid of that pebble. You pick it up, walk towards the water's edge, and throw it far out to sea, as far as you can, so that it is well away from you, right out of your life.

You look back at the other pebbles lying there in the sand and you go over to have a closer look at them, once again realizing what each one represents. Now it seems easier, there is no need to hang onto them any more. As you recognize each one, and decide that you do not need it you place it in a bucket with all the rest. When there are no more pebbles left, you carry the bucket to the water's edge and throw each pebble away, right out of your life.

Soon all the pebbles are gone and you stand there calmly in the water with gentle waves lapping around your feet and ankles. You somehow feel cleansed, feel free, feel able to move forward into a new way of thinking. Now you begin to think of the positive attributes that you want for yourself: love, confidence, happiness, self-esteem—all the things that you ever wanted for yourself and which you know are really your birthright.

You feel that each soft wave that touches your body represents one of these positive emotions. You sense yourself being filled with all the feelings that you ever wanted. As you stand there in the sunshine you feel once again like a child, carefree, happy, ready to join in with the other people on the beach, knowing that you deserve all these good things that you have drawn to yourself.

Spend as much time as you want to on this beach, knowing that you can go back there whenever you wish.

There are two purposes to this fantasy.

• To be aware of negative aspects of yourself and to know that you can let them go. It is only when you can clear your mind of negative thoughts that you can begin to replace them with positive ones.

• To program yourself in a powerful and effective way by showing your subconscious mind, through visualization, what you want for yourself.

Depending on how long you have held the negative thoughts in your mind, you may need to do this exercise a few times before you have completely eradicated the destructive thought patterns.

As you become more confident and adept at using self-hypnosis, you will no doubt develop guided fantasies of your own that are appropriate to you. Keep them simple and above all, enjoy them.

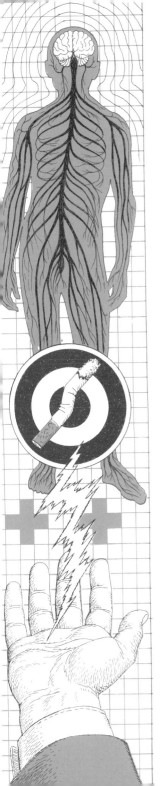

Chapter Six

Developing Personal Programs

Now comes the time when you can adapt our suggestions to suit your specific problems—that is, of course, if you have any problems. We guess, though, that the fact you picked up this book and tape means that you have some area in your life in which you would like to make changes.

The problem areas that we have selected to include in this chapter have been chosen with great care. Not only have we picked out common problems but, more importantly, problems that we know can be successfully dealt with using self-hypnosis. If your problem is not included, refer to Chapter Seven where we detail those problem areas that we think require expert attention. After all our years as practicing hypnotherapists, we believe that some problems—alcoholism, for example—are best tackled in consultation with an experienced therapist.

The text for each of the subjects covered in this chapter is split up into three parts: the affirmation (which includes a "trigger" word), additional exercises, and comments.

• *The affirmation and the trigger word.* An affirmation is a positive suggestion you give yourself that your subconscious mind can understand and act upon. We give you various affirmations, most of which just consist of a few sentences, but of course you can expand on those if you wish in order to suit your own personal circumstances. The length of an affirmation should not be more than five or six sentences. If you make it too long or complicated your conscious mind is likely to come into play and that would negate the benefits of being in hypnosis.

One thing that is important to add onto an affirmation is your own personal reason, or indeed incentive, for wanting to make that change. An example of this might be "Because I want to wear a smaller size dress for my wedding, I now take control of my appetite and I am eating less each day."

As you look at the affirmations, you are no doubt going to start thinking, "I won't be able to remember all that." So, we suggest that before you take yourself into hypnosis you read the affirmation out loud to yourself two or three times, using the word in large bold letters as a "trigger." When you take yourself into hypnosis, you can just say the trigger word and your subconscious mind will automatically run the rest of the affirmation through for you. Did you realize that your subconscious mind was that clever?

• *Additional exercises.* Some of these can be used at the same time as the affirmations or they can be done separately. With some of the longer ones, you may care to record them on to a tape yourself. You probably do not like the sound of your own voice—not many people do—but if you do it yourself, for yourself, then it is much more personal, bearing in mind that you are the person that you trust the most. You will get used to it eventually.

If you do decide to record the exercises on to tape, then do remember to keep your voice to a normal conversational tone. Establish a comfortable rhythm and just speak a little slower than you would normally.

• *Comments.* Our comments are based on our experience of how other people have dealt with their problems. We also include some hints on how you can help yourself in a practical way to achieve what you want in hypnosis.

The instructions for working with the affirmation for Increasing Confidence form the basis of the procedure for all the affirmations in this chapter—it is important to read through this example to find out how to use the other affirmations.

How to Increase Your Confidence
The affirmation

Trigger word: CONFIDENCE

As I relax more and more, I am aware of my own positive resources and therefore I feel more confident.

Each day I feel more positive about myself and realize that I am taking control of my life.

As I become more confident, I know that I can achieve my fullest potential.

I recognize more and more all the good things I have done in my life. I hold my head high as I now feel good about myself.

I have a relaxed attitude towards myself and towards others, and therefore I feel confident when I am with other people.

I have confidence in every situation, I cope well with everything that life has to offer and I enjoy my life to the full.

I now have a positive picture of myself in front of me, looking totally confident, totally in control and totally sure.

Every day I become more aware of my own talents and abilities and my confidence increases more and more.

Having read this aloud to yourself two or three times, including the trigger word, take yourself into hypnosis and allow yourself a little while to relax on your garden bench. Then say the trigger word. You may find some of the phrases running through your mind but rest assured that your subconscious has taken them in and is now acting upon them. As we have said before, the more often you do this, the more powerful it becomes.

You now have a trigger word but you can have a physical trigger as well to help you with your confidence. This is how to acquire one.

When you are in hypnosis, take some time to sit on your garden bench and relax both your body and your mind. Then think of a time and situation in your life when you have felt totally confident. Maybe you think that you have never ever been confident but think again. Perhaps you have felt totally at ease with your close friends, in your work place, or in your own home with your own family. There is certainly at least one situation where you do feel confident. Think of that situation, however simple it might seem—maybe just sitting round a table with your close family. It does not matter what it is, just as long as you can think of it vividly.

Take some time to picture yourself in this situation of feeling fully confident. How do you look when you feel confident? What type of clothing are you wearing? What type of expression do you have on your face? Listen to what you say to others. What tone of voice do you use? What sort of things do you say to yourself when you are feeling confident? How does it feel to be this confident? Where in your body do you have that feeling?

Remember you are doing this in hypnosis and therefore the critical nature of the conscious mind is by-passed. Thinking of that time when you were totally confident, make it even more clear, put all the feeling into it that you can. Experience the emotions that went with it and think to yourself that you are going to make that feeling ten times stronger. Only when you have done that, can you gain a physical trigger.

Here is what you do: you just gently close your right hand. In this way you hold on to that feeling of self-belief and you give a physical trigger to your subconscious mind. Every time you consciously make that physical movement, it will bring back that feeling of complete confidence.

Don't just take our word for it—try it and see for yourself. The more you use it, the better it gets.

Trigger word: COPING

How to Cope with Stress
The affirmation

As I become more relaxed in hypnosis, that relaxation stays with me and I become more relaxed in my daily living.

I know that relaxation is the key to a healthy life and therefore the more I relax the healthier I become.

As my nerves become stronger, I become stronger within myself.

Because I am more relaxed, I cope well with all situations in a very calm way.

All my thoughts are kept in perspective, all my thoughts are positive, therefore I have a new feeling of well-being.

My mind is relaxed, my body is relaxed and I just feel much better about myself.

The more I relax in this way, the more confident I become, the more I can cope beautifully with everything.

I now have a clear picture in my mind of myself and in this picture I cope beautifully with anything. I am totally calm, totally relaxed and totally optimistic.

Additional exercise

When you are really relaxed in hypnosis, really feeling as though you could cope with anything, gently close your left hand. This will help you to hold on to that feeling, that ability to cope, and the more you use it, the more powerful it becomes. You can bring it back at any time during your day to day life by gently closing your left hand again. Do make sure that you always use the same hand. (If you prefer, you can combine this trigger with the one for confidence so that both triggers will be fired by closing your right hand.)

Stress is something of which we are all aware. It is true to say, however, that we are usually only aware of it when we have too much. It could be said that a certain amount of pressure is good for us as it can act as a strong motivator—it is how we cope with it that affects our lives.

If you have ever felt that being completely free from stress would be something to strive for, remember that another word for this condition is death! The word "stress" is often bandied about, and, in this context, is actually being used in place of "harmful stress."

A certain amount of stress is not only desirable but essential. Not only does adrenalin pumping through the body help to bring about better performance such as in acting or interviews but, without it, we would not be able to experience high levels of enjoyment. For example, think about how you get pleasure from say, riding a roller coaster, making love or watching a horror movie.

So, how would we define stress? Of the many definitions around, the one that seems to fit the best goes like this: "Stress is the reaction in an individual's body or mind when that person perceives a potential threat to his or her emotional or physical wellbeing." (*Fight or Flight*, Hughes and Boothroyd 1985.) The operative word here is perceives. If we do not perceive a situation as stressful, then it isn't.

It is not threats that cause stress, that do the damage—stress is created by the body's response to those threats. Here is an example. A young child gets enjoyment from climbing a tree. This activity contains elements of excitement, adventure, danger and so on. Being at the top of the tree, with the wind blowing, can be fun for a child. But now imagine the child's mother. The scenario is likely to be anything but fun for her. She perceives the situation as potentially dangerous so it is likely to be extremely stressful for her. The situation remains the same for both child and mother but it is the mother who feels the stress, not her child.

What actually happens in a stress reaction is extremely complicated. Whenever we feel threatened, either physically or emotionally, our sympathetic nervous system (subconsciously activated) switches on our "fight or flight" response, resulting initially in increased adrenalin levels in the bloodstream. This causes several reactions: the muscles tense up (aches and pains); our digestive system switches off (butterflies in the stomach); the blood is diverted from the skin to the muscular system (paling of the skin); the body's thermostatic system is switched on (sweaty palms and nervous perspiration). In other words, the body prepares either to stand and fight or to run away.

Of course, in the modern world, situations actually requiring a fight or flight response are few and far between. However, because our basic survival instinct is so powerful, we still respond to threat (real or imaginary) in the same way that our prehistoric ancestors did. As we have already said, it is the sympathetic nervous system that instigates the "fight or flight" response but, because nature balances things out, another part of our nervous system is designed to restore our body's equilibrium—the parasympathetic nervous system. For instance, sexual arousal is controlled by the sympathetic nervous system, and orgasm by the parasympathetic nervous system.

Our nervous systems cope admirably with sudden, highly stressful situations and balance is usually restored quickly. But modern life is more subtle—sudden threats are few and far between and we have to deal with persistent pressures—city life, traffic jams, deadlines, advertisements, and so forth. The list goes on and on.

So, when we experience long-term, low-level stress, the battle for equilibrium goes on for far longer than it was originally designed to do, getting more and more fierce, until something gives. If the situation remains, then the sort of thing that may occur is heart attack, stroke, ulcers, depression, anxiety, and cancer. Different people respond to stress in different ways but we do all respond, one way or another.

If, say, you are unhappy in a relationship or with your job and you are suppressing those unhappy feelings because you really feel that you must remain in that situation, then you will experience stress on a subconscious level. If you think that by "putting it out of your mind," you are dealing with it, remember that you are only putting it out of your conscious mind. In other words, you will not be consciously aware of the battle for survival that is going on beneath the surface. Anyone can remain in such a situation for years without realizing the damage that is being done..

In our opinion, most, if not all, physical illness has a psychological element. Medical science seems to be coming more into line with this type of thinking, particularly regarding the part stress plays in illness. High blood pressure, a common ailment in modern society, is often caused by long-term, low-level stress and usually goes undetected. Also, because the stress response has a detrimental effect on the immune system, one indication that stress is present can be a tendency to catching colds, flu and so forth.

For the most part, whenever stress is mentioned, the word "relaxation" is not far behind. And certainly, relaxation in itself is therapeutic. However, when it comes to stress, and we return to the analogy of the automobile, you could say that relaxation techniques for combating the effects are a bit like teaching someone to repair crumpled bodywork after they have hit the wall. We feel that it would be far better to be able to avoid hitting the wall in the first place!

So, to sum up, the stress mechanism is linked

directly to our belief structure, inasmuch as a situation is only stressful if we perceive it to be potentially threatening. Our belief structure is subconscious in nature so, by using hypnosis which is the most direct way to access the subconscious mind, we can adjust our belief structure and alter our response to potentially stressful situations.

How to Control Weight
The affirmation

Trigger words: *SLIM FIGURE*

As I become more relaxed, I realize that I am taking control, control of my appetite and control of my life.

Because I have more respect for myself and my body, I decide to eat only what my body needs.

I know that light, clear, clean foods naturally bring about a light, clear, clean body. I enjoy eating low calorie, healthy foods more and more.

I eat smaller portions, I eat at regular meal times, I am full of satisfaction having taken control in this way.

I constantly see myself as the new slim me, looking fit and healthy, looking slim, looking in control. I hold this picture in my mind of the new me all the time, especially when getting up in the morning, just before going to bed at night, and also just before eating food.

I am really pleased with the way I see myself now and I look forward to the day when the new me merges with this positive picture in reality.

If there is ever a time when I think of food and know for sure that it is not appropriate at that moment, then I just place my hand on my stomach and think to myself, "SLIM FIGURE." That immediately gives me a feeling of inner satisfaction so that I know I don't need to eat.

• This affirmation includes a physical trigger. If you feel hungry at an inappropriate time, you just place your hand on your stomach and think those words *"SLIM FIGURE."*

• In hypnosis, picture the foods that you know you should not be eating if you want to be slim—fattening foods, the sort that you have been eating unnecessarily, and particularly those foods to which you feel you may be addicted. Put this picture in front of you, frame it, and then put a big black cross through it. By doing this, you will give your subconscious mind a direction that those foods are no longer appropriate, no longer necessary.

As you go about your daily life, do not think that you are "losing" weight. Who wants to "lose" anything? Think instead of "achieving" a slimmer figure.

It is true that the only way to weigh less is to eat less but anyone who has ever had a weight problem will know that this is easier said than done because you instinctively know that a part of your mind is stronger than your willpower. That part is of course your subconscious mind and it has its own reasons for keeping you overweight. Until those reasons are established, it is difficult to re-program yourself into eating in a healthy way. Let us look at some of those possible reasons, many of which we frequently encounter in the course of our work with clients.

• Eating to get attention. A good example of this was a client who, having been asked in hypnosis why she was overweight, said that it was to get attention. As she said the words, a quizzical look came over her face and it was obvious that her conscious mind was in conflict with what her subconscious mind was saying. As she reported afterwards, *"I could hardly believe that it was me who was saying that."* However, a quick regression back to childhood revealed that when she was taking part in a school concert, her teacher had said to her, *"You stand in the middle of the stage, because you are the biggest, and then everyone can see you."* Being center-stage appealed to her greatly and her subconscious mind latched onto the idea that if, she was big, then she got noticed. Consequently, her subconscious mind made sure that she stayed big and indeed got bigger and bigger by overeating. No matter how many expensive diets she went on, no matter how many times she lost weight, she would always revert back to her old habits which were to ensure that she stayed "big." Once she became aware of how her subconscious mind had been programmed in this way, then a rapid resolution came about.

• Eating for comfort. An illustration of this syndrome was a very large lady who, when regressed to being four years old, remembered that she was playing in the yard, all on her own, because her elder brother was very ill and everyone else was in the house attending to him. She was feeling bored and neglected. Then she saw some apples lying on the ground, which had fallen off a laden tree, and she decided to eat them. This instantly made her feel better. Her eating program had been well and truly established in those few minutes—in later years, whenever she felt bored or neglected, she ate to give herself comfort again.

• Eating for protection. One lady told us that she had been sexually abused as a child over a period of several years. The thought that kept going through her mind during those years was, "When I am bigger no one will be able to do this to me." Needless to say, she made sure that she got bigger—outwards as well as upwards. She gained weight, lots of it, so that subconsciously she knew that no one would find her sexually attractive and therefore no one would want to have sex with her.

In all these cases, once the reason was known on a conscious level, a change of program in the subconscious mind could easily be made.

Trigger word: *FREEDOM*

How to be Free of Smoking
The affirmation

As I relax more and more, I realize that I do not need to smoke.

I now have a strong desire to be healthy, to have more energy, to be able to breathe easily, to be in control.

As I take control, I am free of cigarettes, free of tobacco, free of nicotine. I am also free to enjoy my life in a healthy way. I am really proud that I am leaving behind an unhealthy, unnatural habit, and know that now I have more respect for my body.

I hear myself refusing cigarettes when they are offered to me and saying to people, "No thanks, I don't smoke."

I enjoy the feeling of freedom that I now have. I enjoy being able to breathe easily, knowing that I no longer smell of tobacco. I know that my teeth are whiter and that I am so much healthier in every way.

The only substitute I need for a cigarette is a long deep breath of fresh air. The more I take that long deep breath, the more relaxed I become and it gives me all the satisfaction that I need.

Every day I am more and more determined to become a non-smoker.

I now have a clear picture of myself as a non-smoker, an ex-smoker, a person who has taken control. I see myself looking healthy, my skin glowing, my hair shiny, my body relaxed, and I look so good.

As you sit on your bench in the imaginary garden that you have created in your mind while listening to the tape, picture that by your side, you can see a pile of cigarettes—a pile of all the cigarettes that you have ever smoked. Those cigarettes are now in the past, they have already gone up in smoke along with the money that you spent on them. Once you have really become aware of just how many cigarettes there are in the pile, then let the picture fade away.

Now decide to place another pile of cigarettes by your side. These represent all the cigarettes that you could smoke in the future if you do not stop smoking right now. You know that you do not really want those cigarettes, do not need them, so now is the time to get rid of these as well. Decide now to make a bonfire of them in the garden. Watch them all burn away, watch the thick black smoke drift away on the breeze away from you, away from your lungs, away from the garden, right out of your life. Watch every last one just turn to ashes.

Now that the last of the smoke has cleared, be aware of the garden again, the fresh, clean air that you can breathe, the freshness of the grass and the flowers, the freshness and cleanliness of yourself.

Each time you do this exercise you are giving your subconscious mind a very definite instruction that cigarettes are now a thing of the past and that that is the way it is going to stay.

Comments

Reprogramming your subconscious mind to get rid of a long-standing habit, an addiction, may take a little while. Most people try to stop smoking using willpower, which means that a large part of their mind, in other words the subconscious, is in conflict with that will power. Usually, when that is the case, people turn to a substitute in the form of extra food, or drugs, or alcohol (what is described as "oral gratification"). However, because you are using hypnosis, you are in touch with that part of your mind that controls your habits and therefore you are much more likely to be successful, no matter how many times you have tried unsuccessfully in the past to quit smoking.

Your attitude of mind, the words you use inside your own head are of prime importance in stopping smoking. For instance, try not to think that you are "giving up" smoking. No one likes to "give up" anything. Think instead about being "free" of a dangerous and unhealthy habit.

There is another trigger which you might find useful when stopping smoking, particularly as most smokers try to find a substitute when they quit cigarettes. More often than not, that substitute is extra food. A much healthier substitute is an extra oxygen intake into your body and you can do that by taking a long deep breath and just saying the word *"FREE-DOM"* to yourself as you breathe out. This becomes both a verbal and a physical trigger, thereby making it twice as strong.

There are several other practical ways you can help yourself while stopping smoking. Some are listed below—choose those which you feel would be most helpful to you.

• Clean your teeth regularly—this keeps your mouth feeling fresh.
• Take a shower more often—it is difficult to smoke in the shower!
• Drink plenty of plain water, six to eight glasses a day. This helps to flush the nicotine and toxins out of your body.
• Always have breakfast as soon as possible after you wake up. This balances your blood sugar level in a natural way, whereas cigarettes boost it in an artificial and unhealthy way.
• Try to avoid all alcohol, tea, coffee and cola. The last three contain caffeine, a stimulant, and they all agitate the nervous system and have a strong associa-

tion with having a cigarette.
• Eat as much fruit and vegetables as you can—these again help to get rid of toxins from the body.
• After a meal (a time which can act as a trigger for a cigarette) go outside (weather permitting), take a walk, and breathe deeply. Try not to sit down in your favorite armchair after a meal or anyplace you always used to smoke a cigarette.
• Take extra vitamins such as B Complex, which is the one that strengthens your nerves, and Vitamin C (you lose Vitamin C when you smoke).
• If you do get that irresistible urge to smoke, stop what you are doing, take a long deep breath and say your trigger word to yourself, remembering that that is your substitute for inhaling tobacco smoke.
• Procrastination is a useful attribute for non-smokers. If that next cigarette can be put off for a while, and then that period extended increasingly, you may never get around to having it! If you think for a moment, you can probably recall a couple of things which you put off for so long, they never got done.

Remember that thousands of people die every year as a direct result of smoking. This causes suffering, not just to the smoker, but also to their loved ones. Also do not forget that many thousands of other people stop smoking every year, some of them after many years, or even decades, of being a smoker. If they can do it, then so can you!

We would also like you to bear in mind that smoking often results because of some emotional need. Ask yourself what it is doing for you.

• Does it relieve stress?
• Does it alleviate worry?
• Does it help you to control your weight?
• Does it help you to stay calm?
• Does it help you to concentrate?
• Does it repress emotions such as anger?

The chances are that you have answered yes to at least one of the questions. In which case, it stands to reason that you should try to find out why you think smoking helps you before trying to quit. In other words, there is no point in trying to remove a symptom if the underlying cause is still there.

Finally, do you want to stop smoking for the right reason? Your motivation must be strong, for instance to improve your health. If you are thinking of stopping smoking just because someone else has advised or nagged you into doing so, then forget it. Wait until you are really doing it for yourself.

Trigger words: *SLEEP WELL*

How to Sleep Well
The affirmation

As I relax more and more during the day, it is only natural that I am more relaxed at night too.

As bedtime approaches, my mind and body relax completely. Thoughts of today or tomorrow just float out of my mind and I feel peaceful and drowsy.

I remind myself that it is my birthright to have a good night's sleep. I remind myself that I am just recapturing something that I used to do easily from the moment I was born: to sleep well and peacefully.

And as I now begin to sleep easily and peacefully throughout the night, then I wake up in the morning fully refreshed and feeling really good about the day ahead.

When I am ready for sleep I have a picture in my mind of myself sleeping peacefully, watching my chest rise and fall, seeing my eyes closed, seeing my body totally relaxed—just sound asleep.

At bedtime, I find it easy to drift from hypnosis straight into a deep and restful sleep.

It would be a good idea to do these two exercises when you go to bed at night.

• Establish yourself on your garden bench and give yourself a definite affirmation that you will go from hypnosis into sleep.

• Imagine that you are drawing a circle up in the sky above those trees surrounding your garden. Above the circle, write the word sleep. Inside the circle, write the number "1." Then very carefully erase that number, making very sure that you do not erase the circle. Then write in the number "2" and so on, until very soon you are fast asleep.

The first sentence in the affirmation is important—first of all because it is true and secondly because it is one that you might not even have considered before. It might be a good idea for you to look at the section on coping with stress and then perhaps combine the two affirmations for optimum effect.

If you are beset with problems in your every day life, then the chances are that you will be taking those problems to bed with you, either consciously or sub-consciously. It is a good idea to keep a notebook by the side of your bed. Make one list of things that have bothered you during the course of the day and a separate list of things that you need to do tomorrow. In this way you are clearing negative thoughts from your mind by writing them down.

If you have had problems sleeping, you will no doubt remember that one of the things you think about as you toss and turn is the fact that you cannot sleep. Hence the reason for the last sentence in the affirmation—it is very important to visualize yourself asleep. We therefore strongly recommend that when you go to bed at night, you take yourself into self-hypnosis and turn your thoughts to something else, something positive, perhaps a pleasant scene in nature or even your own garden with which you will have by now become familiar. Relax your body bit by bit, as you do when listening to the tape.

Remember that if you have been in the habit of taking sleeping pills, then you have just been dealing with the symptom (yes, insomnia is a symptom). By dealing with the stress factors in your life, by dealing with your day-to-day problems in a more positive way, and by learning how to relax properly, the cause of that symptom can be eliminated.

We would also recommend that you examine any possible physical reasons for your insomnia. For instance, if you drink ten cups of coffee a day (taking in an abundance of stimulating caffeine), then there is a good chance that even though your hypnosis might be superb, you will still not sleep. Likewise, if you have a heavy meal late at night, your body will have to work overtime to process the food—if your digestion continues to work long after you have gone to bed, then it might very well keep the rest of your body awake as well.

If you have tried relying on alcohol to help you sleep, you may have realized by now that it might "zonk" you out for a while but very rarely does it provide you with a whole night's sleep or even good quality sleep. Nicotine is a powerful stimulant too, and just to add to all that, there is a great deal of caffeine in ordinary chocolate. Caffeine in either chocolate, coffee, or cola can still be in your bloodstream four or five hours after you have taken it in.

How to Think Positively
The affirmation

Trigger words: *THINK POSITIVE*

As I relax more, I become aware of positive energies within me and around me, and I become more aware of my own inner resources.

I know that as I become more positive in my way of

thinking, I become more positive in my daily life.

I choose to look at everything in a positive way, to think about everything in a positive way, and to experience everything in a positive way.

I allow my mind to open up to accept all that is good and positive in my life. New ideas spring to mind as to how I can improve the quality of my life in every way.

I now forgive myself for any mistakes that I have made in the past, knowing that from those mistakes I can learn and grow.

I look forward to each new day as an opportunity to enjoy and improve my life.

I now have a very clear picture of myself looking positive, looking poised and confident, and I see myself looking this way at all times.

Additional exercise

While in hypnosis, think of some of the negative feelings that you would like to be rid of such as anger, frustration, guilt, and resentment. Realize that you really want all of these feelings to be in the past, that they do not belong to you any more.

Now put all those negative feelings into a box. Put the lid on the box and decide to get rid of it and its contents. You may care to throw it over a cliff into the sea, you may want to bury it in a deep hole, you may care to blow it up, or even set fire to it. Whatever method you choose, make sure that you get rid of it once and for all.

Bearing in mind that those negative thoughts have probably been with you for a long time, it might be a good idea to do this exercise several times as no doubt some of that negativity is deeply entrenched. Each time you do the exercise, feel a little bit lighter, a little bit freer, a little bit more positive, until you know that you have let go of those negative thoughts and are now ready to move forward in a new, positive, and refreshing way.

There are probably hundreds, if not thousands, of books on positive thinking, some of them beautifully written and with some marvellous ideas for thinking in a positive way. But if you are in a negative frame of mind, it is almost impossible to think positively—it is like swimming against a powerful tide that endlessly pushes you back to your starting point..

Willpower alone will not bring about positive thinking; it is essential that the subconscious mind is programmed to think in a positive way as well. So, it seems logical that one of the first steps is to get rid of negative thoughts. Hence the reason for the additional exercise.

Trigger Word: *CLEAR SKIN*

How to Deal with Skin Problems
The affirmation

As I practice my self-hypnosis every day, I have a new relaxed attitude towards myself and towards other people. As I relax more and more, my nerves become stronger and steadier, and my nerve endings become soothed and calm.

As this happens, my circulation improves, particularly the circulation to those blood vessels supplying my skin, and therefore my skin becomes better nourished and healthier. If I ever feel the need to scratch my skin, I am immediately reminded that that is just an old habit, one that I do not need any longer.

The more relaxed I become, the more my skin is soothed and healed, becoming clearer and healthier day by day. It feels more and more comfortable.

My own self-healing processes are now speeding up,

renewing the cells in my body, and especially those cells of the skin.

I now see myself with beautiful, clear skin, just the way i want myself to be. I look fit and healthy, calm and relaxed, glowing with good health.

Additional exercise

Use your imagination as vividly as you can to picture yourself going inside your own body. Have a look at your skin from the inside and establish what work needs to be done by your sub-conscious mind to bring about healing.

You may need to increase the blood supply, or even cleanse it. You may need to do some repair work like scraping or smoothing off. Only you know what work is necessary because only you can see inside your body in this way.

Take it from us that the more you do this work, the clearer the pictures become and, however superficial or strange this may seem to you, do remember that you are giving a direction to your sub-conscious mind (in pictures) of what you want it to do for you.

Comments

There are different kinds of skin problem and each should be treated differently. Mistakes have been made in the past. For instance, people have treated psoriasis in the same way as they have eczema, and vice versa. Psoriasis is often caused by repressed anger. You have no doubt heard the expression "red with anger," so, if anger has not been expressed verbally or physically, then it often erupts through the skin as it has to come out somewhere. However, eczema is usually caused by irritation, sometimes with just one person. Have you ever heard someone say. "He really gets under my skin?"

Hopefully we have made it clear that it is no good just treating a symptom. It would be as well for you first of all to look at the possible causes, starting perhaps with stress.

Trigger word: *EASY BREATHING*

**How to Deal
With Asthma**
The affirmation

As I practice my self-hypnosis, I become calmer and more relaxed in every way.

As my mind becomes more relaxed, my body becomes more relaxed—my bronchial tubes relax, my chest muscles relax, and my breathing becomes easier and easier.

I regularly take long deep breaths, filling my lungs with fresh air, opening up my bronchial tubes, cleansing all my air passages. Each time I do this I feel all tension leaving my body and I feel so comfortable.

My lungs and bronchial tubes and all my air passages are now becoming stronger and clearer, helping me to breathe in a calm and an easy way.

The more relaxed I become, the better I feel and the easier I can breathe, both during the day and night. I feel more comfortable at all times.

I now have a very clear picture of myself looking fit and healthy, breathing easily and naturally and coping with everything in a calm and relaxed way.

I become more and more confident that I am learning to take control of my own body.

Additional exercise

When you are really relaxed and are absolutely sure that your breathing is free and easy, say to yourself the trigger word and lightly place one hand on the top part of your chest. This is a physical trigger for you to use in the future so that if you do have any breathing problems, then each time you place your hand there on your chest, it reminds your body, your bronchial tubes, and all your air passages, of just how free and easy your breathing can be.

Make sure that you always use the same hand and

always place it on the same part of your chest. You will amaze yourself at how effective this can be.

Asthma can have many causes, but the psychological one that we have found to be the most common is what we call part of the "crying syndrome"—in other words, suppressed tears. This can be mixed with anger, or frustration. So, once again, it is important to look at those kind of factors in your life before you start to deal with just the symptom.

Obviously, we cannot ignore the possible environmental causes of asthma. Pollution does play a part, either through pollen in the air, the increased use of the internal combustion engine, through the use of chemical fertilizers sprayed onto crops, through additives in food, and so on. The list could run to pages but it is our objective in this book to look at the psychological causes.

Recent data regarding asthma in children relate that one child in seven now has the disease. This is a frightening thought but, if the causes are solely environmental, then why is it that all children do not have it? The fact is, that one child's immune system is different to another's. Again, maybe we should ask why that is. It could be because of genetic inheritance or the environment. It could also be that one's immune system is affected by how one thinks and by one's emotional development. We strongly believe that the latter explanation is the strongest.

Of course, asthma is not just limited to children. More and more adults are succumbing to it now and this could be because of stress.

So, before you work on the affirmation, look at your lifestyle and pinpoint the stress factors in your life. Ask yourself if you are one of those people who cannot or will not cry. Ask yourself if you are holding in anger—is there something that you want to "get off your chest?"

We have found on occasion that asthma has

occurred because of one specific incident in the past and it has only been possible to isolate that incident through regression work. A case that we dealt with some years ago springs to mind. This was a lady of about thirty-five, when asked in hypnosis if the asthma started when she was young, she regressed to being a child of three. She recalled that, a few days after her mother had returned from hospital with a new baby, she had run into the room where her mother and the new baby were. She was laughing and shouting and about to say something to her mother when all of a sudden her mother shouted at her and told her that the baby was asleep and that she had to be quiet. She gasped with the shock of being scolded and her mood sank from one of elation to one of dejection. That gasp of astonishment, that shock to her system, set off a chain reaction. She continued to gasp whenever she was upset and that eventually developed into a habit until she had full-blown asthma.

How to have an Easy Childbirth
The affirmation

Trigger words: *HAPPY BIRTH*

Because I desire an easy and comfortable childbirth, I now allow feelings of relaxation and increased confidence to become a part of my daily life.

I know that my mind controls my body and as I relax in my mind, my muscles relax in my body.
The time I spend each day in relaxation prepares me for the birth of my baby, making it easier when the time comes to relax and enjoy a natural birth.

Each day in relaxation, I talk to my baby and tell it everything it needs to know, reassuring it and preparing it for this wonderful event.

As the time of birth draws near, and the contractions begin, I welcome them, being aware of them, and know-

ing that each one is a step nearer to my baby being born I find that the contractions do not bother me because I am so relaxed and comfortable.

I remind myself daily that everything I experience is a totally natural event and so I look forward to the future, to the new life growing inside me, and to the new life to be shared with my baby.

Additional exercise

When you have practiced your self-hypnosis for several days and you are really proficient at achieving a relaxed state, you can give yourself a physical trigger that you can use during the actual delivery.

So, only when you feel that you have one hundred per cent relaxation, gently stroke your stomach with your hand. Tell yourself that your stroking immediately brings comfort, relaxation and a feeling of total control.

If you want to involve your husband or partner in this, you can give the suggestion that, as he strokes your stomach or indeed your back, you will receive that same feeling.

This does not mean to say that you will not feel the contractions. It is important that you do feel them so that you can assist in the birth but you do not have to feel them with pain.

Comments

The expectation that childbirth has to be painful is due in no small measure to "old wives' tales." For countless generations, negative programming has been passed on from mother to daughter, friend to friend, and has become part of our culture. That is why it is vital that preparation for, and knowledge of, the birth process is given during pre-natal care.

It is a fact that our bodies can produce their own chemicals to block pain. These are endorphins and enkephalins which share the same chemical properties as morphine. Because we are using hypnosis, and therefore accessing the subconscious mind which facilitates the activity of these natural painkillers, we are able to encourage their production.

It is also a fact that tension certainly aggravates, and often causes, pain. By helping yourself to relax, and thereby convincing yourself that you can take control and that childbirth is a natural process, you are half way to establishing a state of mind where you know that childbirth can be a trouble-free event. Indeed, it can be and should be a joyous occasion.

Research carried out in England by Drs. Jenkins and Pritchard found that women using hypnosis in their first pregnancies achieved a significant reduction in the duration of the first stage of labour. In addition, a significant proportion of women using hypnosis required no chemical anesthesia in the later stages. This was reported in the *British Journal of Obstetrics and Gynaecology* in March 1993.

Another important benefit of using hypnosis for pain relief, rather than conventional painkillers, is that the baby cannot be hurt or damaged in any way by chemical anesthetics. Until a baby is born, it receives all its nourishment and oxygen from its mother. If these life-giving supplies are contaminated with anesthetics, then it is likely that they will reach the baby—not a good start to life outside the womb. Also, of course, the mother remains fully able to respond to the instructions of the midwife or doctor and can participate fully throughout delivery because she is fully conscious..

How to Increase Your Spirituality
The affirmation

Trigger word: *SPIRITUALITY*

I am now opening up my mind to accept and enjoy all that is good and wonderful in this universe of which I am a part.

I am entitled to receive the light and the love which is in abundance around me. It is my birthright and therefore I deserve it.

I constantly think of drawing to myself a golden light and then spreading that light out to everyone I meet.

I become more and more aware of the beauty of creation as well as the loving energy within me and in all other people.

I trust in my Higher Self and recognize that I have a constant guiding presence within me.

I am a child of the universe, I am a part of that wonderful creation, and I constantly seek to see the good in all things.

Additional exercise

Once again, find yourself seated on your garden bench, looking around at all the beautiful things in nature—the trees, the flowers, the grass, and the vastness of the sky. Allow yourself to be in harmony with your surroundings.

As you look at the sky, imagine that you are being transported upwards in a golden bubble, rising slowly, easily and naturally, as if being lifted by some unseen hand. Just float steadily upwards, away from the garden and up into the vastness of the blue sky.

Continue floating higher and higher until the garden below you becomes just a small speck in the distance. Feel a sense of security and wonderment; feel uplifted as you are carried into what seems a timeless existence, higher and higher.

Warm and comfortable in your golden bubble, look at the stars, shining more brightly than you have ever seen them, as the sky grows darker. See a particular star, one that is surrounded by a golden light, and realize that you are moving closer and closer towards it. The star seems like a place that you have visited before and you are eager to arrive at your destination.

Your bubble brings you safely down onto the star and you are deposited gently on the ground outside a domed, white building. This building seems familiar and is surrounded by the most beautiful gardens.

Walk up to the open doors of the building and enter. Again you are surrounded by a golden glow and you gaze around in wonderment. There is a feeling of perfect peace and tranquillity. In the center of the room that you are now standing in, there is a chair which somehow you know is there just for you.

Walk over to the chair, sit down and wait. You have an air of expectancy and feel comfortable and safe. An archway at the far end of the room catches your attention and there, framed in it, is the figure of a person whom you seem to recognize—a person who gives you a welcome feeling of being home, someone you know you can trust completely.

You feel love, light and warmth emanating from this person. Everything seems so natural, like distant memories of something that you have experienced before, a long time ago. As the figure moves closer to you, you know that there is no need for words, the communication is already there.

You know that you are going to ask a question about your life's purpose and you instinctively know that this guiding presence will be able to answer—perhaps in words, perhaps just with a feeling, or even a picture. Ask the question that is uppermost in your mind and wait for the answer.

You are reminded that this person has always been a part of you, has been there to guide you and will always be there for you. Stay in this wonderful place for a while and enjoy the peace, tranquillity and loving warmth. Now that you have found the way, know that you can come back at any time you wish.

After a while, return to your own surroundings, to the place where you belong on earth. Be guided gently back in your golden bubble, back through that timeless zone, always surrounded by that golden light, back to your garden once again. Bring with you that feeling of harmony with your Higher Self and that knowledge that can help you continue your life's journey.

It has been said that hypnosis is the gateway to prayer. Let us look at this in a logical way.

First of all, we have a conscious mind, which is the one we are aware of using most of the time. Secondly we have a subconscious mind, which by now you are probably getting to know quite well. And thirdly, we have what could be described as a superconscious mind or, as some would describe it, our Higher Self, our link to divine or cosmic consciousness, or even our soul. Whichever way you want to think about it is right for you and we certainly do not intend to be dogmatic in our views on this as everyone finds their own level, either in hypnosis or in their every day way of thinking.

However, as we approach the new millennium, it is very much apparent that thousands, if not millions, of people are searching for that elusive "something else," that enlightenment, that spark of divine power, that connection with something we know is there but do not quite know where to find.

Most people look in the wrong places. They search outside themselves, travelling from one guru to another to find the secret of life, whereas we firmly believe that enlightenment is within each and every one of us.

If enlightenment is inside us already, what better way to find it than through the channel that you have already begun to travel along, in other words through hypnosis and through your very own subconscious mind?

You know from reading previous parts of this book that one definition of hypnosis is an "altered state of consciousness," so from that altered state, it must be relatively easy to move on to the next one. Use the affirmation, and the additional exercise, to instruct your subconscious mind as to what you want and employ them to find your Higher Self. As is so often the case, success comes with practice—persevere and you will get there.

How to Improve Your Memory
The affirmation

Trigger Words: *GOOD MEMORY*

Everything that I have experienced is stored in my sub-conscious mind. Therefore, as I become more relaxed, I become more confident in my ability to recall all the details that I need.

The more relaxed I am, the more I open up the channel to my subconscious mind and the easier it is to access information quickly and accurately.

With each day that passes, I relax more and more. In this way I am able to recall facts and figures better than ever before—I just relax and let my mind work efficiently for me, helping me to concentrate and recall with ease.

I am confident that I can rely on my memory to give me all the facts I need, as and when I need them. I now enjoy the benefit of perfect recall.

As I relax in this way, I am allowing my conscious and subconscious minds to work together as a team for my benefit.

Additional exercise

Once you are sitting on your garden bench and you have relaxed your mind, decide to double your relaxation, maybe by using the ruler technique that we described in Chapter Five. Take yourself down to your optimum level of relaxation.

Once there, at a level with which you feel comfortable, imagine vividly that you are going inside your own head to find the memory channel which links your conscious to your subconscious mind. You may see it as a tube or a pathway—whatever seems right to you is fine. Check that the memory channel is cleared to accept the information you want to retrieve. You may see debris there or obstacles of some sort—whatever it is, just clear it out of the way and give a very strong instruction to your subconscious mind that you only want positive memories to be recalled.

This is a strong and powerful visualization, so make sure that you are specific. Remember, that the subconscious mind hides certain memories for our own benefit—we would literally go crazy if we could remember everything that had ever happened to us. It is also worth realizing, if you have not done so already, that the subconscious mind has its own logic—memories are often recalled as objects or even as images.

Comments

There is a common misconception about memory. If we have problems in remembering facts and figures, more often than not we will say things like, "I have a terrible memory" or "I have no memory for ..." In actual fact, our memory is perfect—it is just the recall that is not so good.

Like so many negative statements, the more we say those kind of things to ourselves, the more we confirm our inability to remember—in effect, such phrases become self-fulfilling prophesies. Have you ever noticed how effortlessly you learn and remember details about subjects that interest you? On the other hand, like most of us, you probably struggle to describe events that you found boring.

There are people who claim that they have no difficulty in memorizing facts or indeed recalling them. Until, that is, they come under pressure—in an examination hall, for example. Then their minds go blank. This is why it is as well to heed the advice often given to students taking exams: answer the easy questions first. This gets students into recall mode rather than non-recall mode and complete panic. Most of you can probably remember a time when you have sat chewing your nails over an examination paper, the elusive answers just not making themselves known to you. Finally, after leaving the examination hall and after you have started to relax, hey presto, like the wave of a magic wand, all the answers you wanted flood into your brain. Would it not have been better to have relaxed before and during the examination? Self-hypnosis could have helped!

While on that subject of studying, it is a good idea to go into hypnosis before you start work. Give an instruction to your subconscious mind to concentrate on your study for a set time, one hour, say, and spend five minutes or so in hypnosis just relaxing your mind and body before you start.

In conclusion, we would say that the more you practice these techniques, and the more relaxed you become, then the quicker you will be able to access any necessary information that you need at a given time. Once you realize how well this new ability works for you, you will become more comfortable with it and you will become more efficient at using it.

How to Heal Yourself
The affirmation

Trigger word: *HEALTHY BODY*

As I allow myself to relax, all the muscles in my body also relax.

This relaxation brings with it a feeling of inner comfort, soothing, calming and repairing every part of me.

This relaxation enables me to be healthier and fitter in every way, allowing my own healing energies to flow more freely.

The more relaxed I become, the more my mind and body work together in harmony with each other, strengthening my immune system, calming my nerves, revitalizing every cell in my body.

I now begin to feel better about myself and better within myself, knowing that my new positive attitude helps to bring about good health.

The more positive I am in my way of thinking, the more my subconscious mind helps me to bring about renewed good health.

I now have a very clear picture in my mind of how I want myself to be. I look fit and healthy and relaxed—just glowing with good health. I bring this picture to my mind constantly to remind myself of exactly what I want for myself.

Additional exercise

Take yourself to your optimum level of hypnosis on your ruler and imagine very vividly that you are going to that part of your body that requires attention. Go right inside and study the section that needs to be repaired, replaced, or whatever. Allow your subconscious mind to give you ideas as to what needs to be done.

Let us say right away that you need absolutely no anatomical or physiological knowledge whatsoever to do this work. Remember that your subconscious mind works in pictures and symbols a great deal—it will give you the appropriate image in a symbolic form and you can work with that.

It is sometimes easier to think of the part that needs repair as being outside your body. You can work on it at your kitchen table or your work bench. However you do it, and however strange it might seem at first, rest assured that it is all right—your subconscious mind will understand what you are doing. If you are working with bones, you may need to smooth things out, to oil the joints. If you are working with muscles, you may need to cool the area down, warm it up, or increase the blood supply. If you are working with the internal organs you may need to repair tissues or take bits away. If you really let go, and go along with the process, you will amaze yourself at the insight you get, the pictures you create, and the results you achieve.

It is important to carry on with the work regularly.

One day, you will "go inside" and know that everything is looking normal and that the healing work is finished.

Comments

There is one fact that we always like to mention when talking to people about the healing aspects of hypnotherapy—the mind and body can heal themselves. Remember that your subconscious mind works automatically every minute of every day to keep you healthy and it is imperative to know that it is normal to be healthy.

An important point that we would like to make, however, is that using hypnosis to heal yourself should not be a substitute for visiting your doctor and getting a medical diagnosis.

Trigger word: *ABUNDANCE*

How to Draw Abundance to Yourself
The affirmation

As I relax more, I allow everything to flow more naturally. I realize that I deserve all the good things that life has to offer.

The more I relax, the more I allow creative ideas to come into my mind that will enrich my life.

There is an abundance of everything that I want on this earth and I am entitled to a share of that abundance.

I value my own talents and abilities. I value my own success. I value the right that I have to receive and to share in the abundance of life.

I use all my resources to the full to bring abundance to myself.

I now open up and accept that wealth can come to me and that I can use it in a proper and generous way for the benefit of myself and others.

Sitting on your garden bench, make a vivid mental picture of one or more specific things that you want for yourself which would show you that you have received abundance. Be specific with this picture, putting in all the details that you can think of.

When you have a clear and attractive picture, draw a large bubble around the items so that the things you want are protected. Now let the bubble be carried off into the far reaches of universal consciousness, wherever you perceive it to be, until you feel that the bubble has made a connection.

After waiting for a while, picture one or more of those things that you want coming back to you and visualize them being placed in the exact space and time where you wish them to be. Feel yourself enjoying them, appreciating them. Finally, thank the universe for giving them to you.

Comments

This might be one of the most difficult exercises for you to do in the whole of this book. Although abundance is often what most of us want in one way or another, it is often the hardest thing to work for because so many of us do not really feel that we deserve it, being reminded of the starving millions in Africa, the beggars on the streets, and so on. In addition, your conscious mind will probably find the concept of being able to receive abundance through the use of self-hypnosis irrational. Your subconscious mind will not be so bothered, however, and it is the subconscious that is being addressed.

It is important to remind yourself that there is an abundance of all things and that each one of us is just as entitled to receive it as the next person. Rest assured that if you are not ready for it, then plenty of other people are.

When working with the affirmation it is vital to reprogram your mind in a new and positive way, to remind yourself over and over again that you actually do deserve abundance.

How to Improve at Sports
The affirmation

Trigger words: *SPORTS SUCCESS*

As I relax more and more each day, I become more fully aware of the skills that I have, the skills that enable me to excel at sports.

Each day I feel more positive about myself, more confident in my abilities, and this shows more and more when I play ....(sport of your choice).

I know that the key to performing well in sports is the ability to relax and let things flow naturally. Through regular practice and regular relaxation, I am able to go with the flow of play with minimum effort and maximum pleasure.

I now see myself playing just as I want to. I notice how I look when I play well, the kind of things I say to myself, the tone of voice I use, and the way I feel inside. I keep this positive picture in my mind at all times. My game improves steadily as each day goes by, and flows just as I picture it.

As I allow myself to go with the flow, my ability to concentrate also increases, enabling me to focus my entire attention on the game when required.

Additional exercise

Once you are in good quality hypnosis, have a clear picture of yourself performing just the way that you would like. If you have any difficulty with this to start off with, then model yourself on your favorite professional player instead.

Either way, imagine things going just how you would like them to go. Study the game in great detail. Notice how that successful person in the picture looks, how they perform, what they say to themselves when they play well, what tone of voice they use, how they actually feel when playing. Take your time to get into the scenario—watch it and feel it. If you choose to put someone other than yourself in the picture, imagine that you take the place of that professional, playing exactly the way that they do, in fact even better. See yourself achieving the desired result and notice how you feel.

When you are really sure that you have accomplished what you want, give yourself a physical trigger, perhaps similar to the one mentioned in the section on confidence. In other words, gently close your left or right hand (if you are right-handed, then that is normally the better hand to choose). As you close your hand in this way, you "hold onto" those positive feelings of success.

Comments

If you think that using hypnosis to improve at sports is something new, then think again. As long ago as 1956, the Soviet Olympic team were accompanied by no less than eleven hypnotists and the Soviet Union won more medals than any other nation, that Olympic year. The coaches obviously recognized the power of the mind and the difference it can make to sports achievement!

However, it must be said that, even if you use the most powerful of self-hypnosis techniques, there is no point in having confidence without competence. But, regular practice coupled with strong visualization techniques and the affirmation given above will give you a head start over your competitors.

Sports professionals confirm that frequent practice is important, not only to improve skills but to make movements "second nature." Successful sports people often visualize each part of their game just prior to playing and this gives their subconscious mind a positive picture of the desired outcome. In addition, they regularly use physical triggers—tennis players and the like often clench their fists after winning a point. This fuels the imagination to go on and do the same again.

Some individuals go through routines or rituals before starting to play. If anything disturbs the ritual, then they usually start all over again. This is also a kind of physical trigger and it needs to be enacted before play begins.

So, why just let the professionals employ the "tricks of the trade?" Personalize the affirmation to suit your own individual game and combine it with the additional exercise to acquire the same "mind set" that is required of all the top sporting personalities.

How to Relieve Pain
The affirmation

Trigger word: COMFORT

As my relaxation increases more and more, then my level of comfort also increases, comfort in mind and body.

As I continue relaxing in this way, I allow myself to let go of anything that has bothered me in the past. I give myself permission to feel easy and comfortable at all times.

I realize that as I take control of my mind, I also take control of my body in a new and positive way.

Relaxation and comfort go hand in hand, and I now allow myself to be filled with good, positive feelings about myself.

The increase in relaxation also allows my healing energies to flow more freely so that they work powerfully to restore balance and harmony within myself.

I now have a clear picture of those healing energies flowing through my body. I see them as a colours, travelling to any part of my body that needs them. They convey relief, warmth, comfort, healing, and a wonderful feeling of wellbeing.

Additional exercise

When you are in hypnosis, turn your attention to the area of discomfort. How does it look? What color is it? What is it shaped like? What size is it?

What color should it be? What color would you like it to be? Change the color, making sure that it is completely different and that no trace of the original color remains.

What size should it be? What sort of shape? Change these as well, if needs be. Notice how easy the area feels, how comfortable it can be. Notice how easy it is to take control and enjoy the feelings of comfort and relaxation.

Comments

Please note: Do not, under any circumstances, remove pain without first knowing its purpose. Pain, often thought of as a problem, is actually a symptom, a signal. If we return to the analogy of the automobile for a moment, imagine you are driving along the road and the oil warning light comes on. Simply removing pain is a bit like removing the oil warning bulb on the assumption that this will enable you to continue your journey.

While it is true that western medicine seems intent on tackling symptoms and removing them, do not remove any yourself without ascertaining from your doctor whether it is safe to do so.

If it is deemed all right to proceed, you might be interested to know that, by using hypnosis to control pain, you are actually prompting the body to produce endorphins, natural painkillers that are many times more effective than morphine.

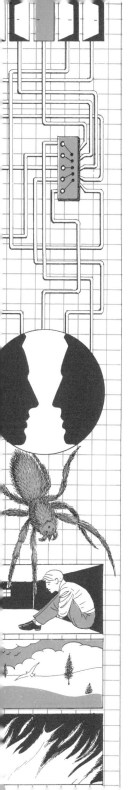

Chapter Seven

Next Steps

It is now time for assessment. No doubt you are becoming quite proficient at using your self-hypnosis techniques and maybe this is the time when you want to experiment and move on to more and more ambitious objectives. But hold on for a minute.

Whereas we have said that there are really are no limits as to what you can do with your own mind, some things are just best left to the professionals. You would not want to attempt to do head surgery on yourself, would you? Well, hypnotherapists, and indeed psychotherapists, psychologists and psychiatrists, use the word "abreaction" to describe an adverse reaction. This can occur when a painful memory comes to the surface.

If you have followed our guidelines so far, there is no way that you can suffer an abreaction, but if you should attempt to do intensive therapy on yourself, then we cannot guarantee the outcome. For instance, you might have thought that you could do a regression (taking yourself back in time in order to uncover hidden feelings or emotions) on yourself, or even a past life regression, in which case, we would say right here and now forget it. This could be highly dangerous. Clear enough?

If a regression of any sort is called for, in other words if you feel that you have unresolved business from the past, then for heaven's sake consult an expert who is a qualified hypnotherapist.

You have already been shown some techniques for how to lose weight and stop smoking, and those techniques are usually extremely effective. But, let us suppose that there is some sort of subconscious blockage in your mind, some reason why your subconscious is firmly convinced that you should hang onto these bad habits, then you should consult a qualified hypnotherapist to help you resolve the situation.

If you have a physical problem, then do not work on it with self-hypnosis until you have had a diagnosis from your doctor. For instance, it would be possible to alleviate a headache using hypnosis, but if it was a brain tumor that was causing that headache, then you would not be doing yourself any favor by getting rid of the symptom.

Although we cannot stress enough how effective hypnosis is, please do not use it as a substitute for obtaining a medical opinion or treatment.

You may wonder why we have not covered a particular problem in the last chapter. There might be a very good reason. We could have forgotten it or, much more likely, we have omitted it on purpose—we firmly believe some problems are best dealt with by a qualified hypnotherapist. But, do not despair—practice your self-hypnosis techniques anyway, certainly to increase your confidence and so on. When you are ready for more dynamic and intensive therapy, you will be better equipped for hypnotherapy and your therapist will find the job easier because you are already proficient at self-hypnosis.

In the next section we will be looking at specific and dynamic techniques employed by advanced hypnotherapists, but in the meantime let us have a look at some of the problems that we feel are best dealt with by an expert.

• *Alcoholism.* This is now regarded by most medical people as being a disease, that is, it is not a weakness. It is not a case of overindulgence and it is certainly not a case of telling someone that they are naughty and should pull themselves together. Alcoholism is a complex matter to deal with, requiring a great deal of understanding and support, and should certainly be left to the professionals. Having said all that, there is no doubt that using self-hypnosis techniques for, say, increasing confidence, would be highly beneficial for the alcoholic, in addition to seeking professional help.

• *Anorexia and bulimia.* These are both life-threatening problems and, because the self-image of the person is usually totally different to the way people see her (we say her because this is usually a problem suffered by girls or young women), then there would be no point in her suggesting to herself in self-hypnosis that she should see herself as the way she really wanted to be! That would just be reinforcing her actual physical condition and would, in effect, make the problem worse, not better.

• *Depression.* If the depression is long-standing, there needs to be an analytical approach to find out why the depression started in the first place and why it has continued. It is important to emphasize here that we are talking about genuine clinical depression and not those feelings that we all have from time to time of just feeling "down." If the depression is of a temporary kind, one that could be called "reactive"—in other words, you feel down because of certain things that have happened—then some of the techniques that we have given you for confidence and for dealing with stress would once again be useful.

• *Phobias.* Here we are talking about real phobias, totally irrational fears of things that most other people cope with quite adequately. The most common phobias that hypnotherapists deal with are agoraphobia (fear of open spaces) and claustrophobia (fear of enclosed spaces). Fear of spiders is another phobia that we frequently come across. There is a reason for every phobia, and once the reason has been established, usually through regression work, then it automatically comes about that the phobia vanishes. This type of work can only be done by a competent therapist but we would say again that you can prepare yourself for working with a hypnotherapist by learning self-hypnosis techniques first, as this will help you to be calmer and more able to cope.

• *Psychosis.* It is almost irrelevant to insert this paragraph as the chances of a psychotic actually picking up this book are negligible. A neurotic knows that there is something wrong with them, a psychotic doe not. Real mental illnesses such as psychosis, schizophrenia, and manic depression, are obviously best dealt with by a psychiatrist.

Although we strongly recommend that you seek expert help if you suffer from one of the problems listed above, we believe that virtually everybody can benefit enormously from self-hypnosis in a very powerful and positive way, even if it is just used to gain confidence in taking the next step.

The Role of the Hypnotherapist
How to find a good hypnotherapist

The safest way of ensuring that you choose a reputable therapist is to follow up on a recommendation either from someone you know who has had therapy and been satisfied with it, or from your own doctor.

Failing that, we would strongly advise you to do the following:

• Look up a name in the telephone directory—there are plenty of them! Single out a person with letters after their name.

• Telephone the therapist and ask what the letters stand for. Also find out how long they have been a hypnotherapist and ask if they would mind you checking their credentials with the organization to which they belong.

• Ask for an initial consultation which places you under no obligation—most ethical therapists offer thi anyway. This first consultation gives you the chance to find out about each other and enables you to determine how comfortable you feel with the therapist. If you have any doubts or uncertainties at all, do not proceed with the therapy. It is vital that you feel you have a good rapport with anyone who is proposing to help you make important life changes.

• Find out how much the therapist charges and how many sessions they think will be required. If the therapist suggests that you pay a large sum up front, say, for a block of sessions, then find another therapist.

As we have already mentioned, the role of the hypnotherapist is crucial for resolving long-standing and firmly entrenched problems, and for helping to remove subconscious blockages.

If a hypnotherapist tells you that he or she can "cure you" then find another therapist. But, if you are told that the hypnotherapist can help you to help yourself, then you can probably work well together.

So, if you decide to consult a hypnotherapist, what kind of techniques and different therapies can you expect to encounter? Let us have a brief look at some of these.

Types of Therapy
Suggestion therapy

This is basically the original form of hypnotherapy and is now regarded by most modern and well trained hypnotherapists as being rather old-fashioned. However, it is the form of hypnotherapy to which the general public relates the most. Most people going to see a hypnotherapist for the first time expect to sit in a chair or lay down on a couch, be put into a trance or a deep state of unconsciousness, and then be told what to do, or not to do, as the case may be. No one can be made to do anything in hypnosis that they do not want to do, and the subconscious mind is very resistant to change, so, before it will make the necessary changes, it needs to realize why.

Now, the whole point of making suggestions/affirmations to yourself in self-hypnosis is that you are the one that is giving yourself the suggestions. Only you know exactly what you want for yourself.

Suggestion Therapy can be usefully employed by a

hypnotherapist as an adjunct to more dynamic therapy and for conditioning the subconscious mind into making changes in the future. However, as you can do this kind of therapy quite well for yourself, then we would suggest that you steer clear of a hypnotherapist who employs only this method.

Aversion Therapy

This form of therapy was used a great deal in the 1940s and earlier. However, most ethical hypnotherapists now realize that it can cause problems for the client—and that a client can actually be made to feel ill—if a suggestion like "every time you smoke you will feel sick" is given.

It is our firm belief that it should be the priority of every hypnotherapist to make a client feel "good" rather than suggesting that they will feel ill if they do a certain thing.

The idea behind Aversion Therapy was that a "state of anxiety" connected with a specific thing should be deliberately invoked, the theory being that the client would then no longer wish to expose himself to that particular stimulus. In other words, it was thought that the client would avoid carrying out the original behavior pattern because he knew that the effects of it would affect him adversely!

Alcoholics, for instance, were often treated with Aversion Therapy, sometimes in addition to drugs administered by a psychiatrist—each time a client drank alcohol, he would be sick. The idea was that he would learn to associate drinking with being sick. In other cases, he would be given an electric shock when drinking, and again the idea was that he would then associate drinking with the effects of the shock. This might seem a rather primitive, if not a barbaric, way of dealing with alcoholics and obviously does not take into account the actual cause of the problem.

Aversion Therapy was based on the notion that when someone is punished for their behavior, then that behavior will be eliminated. Modern thinking now works on the basis that behaviour changes are more likely to take place if someone is rewarded for good behaviour, rather than punished for bad. Thankfully, Aversion Therapy has largely been superseded by more up-to-date methods and would now never be used by an ethical hypnotherapist.

Recently, Ann, a woman in her mid-thirties, came to us regarding a weight problem. She explained that she had been for a course of hypnotherapy a few years ago and was concerned about repeating that experience. It transpired that her original therapist had worked with visualization techniques and had asked her to imagine that she was going along a dark tunnel where there were sharp knives. Not only was this ineffective, but it was distressing for the client.

Our belief is that people have got problems enough, without the therapist adding on to them!

Regression Therapy

This is often the type of therapy that first of all interests a client most but then brings about the most fear. It seems to be a fascination for most people to want to go back, either to an earlier time in this life, or for an increasing number of people, back to an earlier lifetime—a "past life regression."

As far as the latter is concerned, it is our belief that this should not be done just for idle curiosity. But there is no doubt that it has been found to be useful in a therapeutic way for certain people, especially if they were convinced that nothing in this lifetime could have affected them so badly!

A typical example of this was a businessman who came for therapy because he had a fear of knives. This was affecting his life very badly as he often had to take important clients out for lunch. At first, no reason for this phobia could be found in hypnosis, but when he was asked if it was the result of a past life experience, he immediately said yes. A past life regression was carried out during which it was ascertained that he had been a merchant in the eighteenth century, and while travelling on horseback one day, he had been accosted by a highwayman who had demanded his money and then stabbed him with a knife, a dagger to be precise.

Whether that actual event was true or not does not really matter because from that time on the man was cleared of his phobia and had no further problems with knives.

There has been a huge increase over the last few years of so-called "experts" specializing in past life regression. Unfortunately, some of these people have not had any training in hypnotherapy and could be doing untold damage to their clients. So, if you wish to experience a regression, you are strongly recommended to consult a competent hypnotherapist who has an expertise in this area of work.

As for regression in this lifetime, one school of thought is that one must find the cause to find the cure. That was probably the case at one time but with the advent of Neuro-Linguistic Programming (more about this later), it is now clear that this is not strictly true. However, it is often more interesting, enlightening, and satisfying to find out the cause of a problem and to realize how it all started.

Again, this type of work should only be done by a competent hypnotherapist who can work through the regression, help the client to assimilate the knowledge gained, and is able to understand the impact that a particular event has had on the client's life since.

Regression Therapy works on the basis that every single thing that has ever happened to us is stored in our memory, in our subconscious mind. For our own sake, our sanity as much as anything else, many of these memories have been locked away, or buried, deep within our subconscious mind, and it is not necessary for us to remember them. Certainly, traumatic memories will have been buried away, for our own protection, and the only time that we need to retrieve them is when they are still causing a problem. The only effective way that this can be done is through hypnosis. Hypnosis opens up the memory channel to the subconscious mind, in a safe way, so that troublesome events can be looked at again through the eyes of an adult rather than with the emotions of a child.

We recently carried out an example of this type of work with a lady in her early forties who came to us wishing to lose weight. Her doctor had advised drastic action as she was continuing to put on weight, which aggravated her asthma, and her life was considered to be at risk. She had tried just about every diet going but, after some initial success, always slipped back into her old eating habits. Merely telling her subconscious that she would eat less would not have had any long term beneficial effect. The cause needed to be found.

In hypnosis, she regressed to the death of her sister to whom she was very close. This event would have been tragic enough but it emerged that, just prior to the death, they had had a major disagreement and were no longer on speaking terms. In hypnosis, the unfinished business with her sister was dealt with and we also took the opportunity to see if her asthma was connected to this in some way. As a result, her asthma cleared up immediately and her weight has reduced steadily, without the need to diet.

Inner child work

We have decided to give a quick mention of this here because, although it is not strictly a part of hypnotherapy, it has been found to be of immense use, particularly following regression therapy. Most of our present day problems relate to incidents or conditions in childhood, so when regression has been done, it is useful to comfort that inner child, reassure it that it has survived, and so on.

Neuro-Linguistic Programming (NLP)

With its dynamic techniques, NLP has advanced hypnotherapy enormously, enabling clients to take full responsibility for enhancing the quality of their lives.

It was devised by two Americans, John Grinder (a linguist) and Richard Bandler (a mathematician), and was based mostly on the work of Milton Erickson and Virginia Satir, and also to a certain extent on the work of Fritz Perls who specialized in Gestalt Therapy.

NLP is in fact centered on a statement by Erickson: "All patients have within themselves the necessary storehouse and reserves to permit change."

NLP enables people to make the correct choices and to develop their own powers of excellence. Over the years, NLP has been used not only in therapeutic situations, but also in the fields of business, education and sport.

The use of NLP is based on the idea that the subconscious mind works like a computer, in other words that the subconscious is programmed from childhood to act, and react, in certain ways in certain situations, and that once a program has been firmly established, it is very difficult to change. However, with the use of hypnosis combined with NLP, those old programs and old conditionings can be changed very rapidly once the subconscious mind has come to realize that the change is beneficial.

The concept of choice is crucial to NLP—it gives people choice when they may previously have thought there was no choice at all. This enables a client, not only to model himself on someone else he admires, but also to model himself on himself, on the past triumphs and successes he has had and on the way he has dealt well with situations in the past.

Also important to NLP is the fact that most people achieve way below their potential. NLP helps them to define what they really want and then to use their inner resources to achieve it.

NLP shows someone how he can actually switch consciousness, from viewing himself as others would see him to how he feels about himself. He can then view those two experiences together. It is an extremely powerful way of gathering information about ourselves.

Sometimes, one session of NLP is all that is needed. A young businessman recently came in at the eleventh hour with a problem involving his work. He was due to give a presentation to some prestigious clients in three days time and realized that, because of the way he was feeling, it just would not be possible. As time was short, a full program of hypnotherapy was not feasible and some immediate first aid was called for.

By using hypnosis and NLP, the client was able to model himself on a television celebrity whom he visualized giving the presentation. As part of the process, he assumed the character of that celebrity and gave the presentation just as he would. On the day of the presentation that is exactly how it went and the client talked with ease and confidence.

HypnoHealing

This was devised by Bill Atkinson-Ball in the early 1960s, first and foremost to deal with his own injuries after an aerial accident in the Royal Air Force.

HypnoHealing works on the basis that the mind heals the body. If we can accept the concept of psychosomatic illness, then surely we can accept psychosomatic "wellness." Most people now accept that if the mind is at "dis-ease," then sooner or later the body will have disease.

The HypnoHealing technique works first of all on eliciting from the subconscious mind whether there is any "secondary gain" for a client's illness—in other words, what subconscious advantages there might be for being unwell—and then removing that blockage and following up with strong visualization techniques. It is important that the visualization is the client's own—it is essential that the client has total freedom to "see" the diseased parts of the body in his own way and then to find ways in which to change those internal pictures in whatever way he thinks fit.

The Simontons in America did a great deal of work in this way although they did not use formal hypnosis.

Working with terminally ill people, they suggested to patients what visualization they should have, sometimes suggesting things like piranha fish or sharks eating up cancer cells.

A lady in her early forties sought hypnotherapy in order to help her become a non-smoker. She arrived for the second session in considerable pain and explained that she had sustained a neck injury at work, resulting in an extended leave of absence. Her worry was that, because of the pain, she would not be able to relax sufficiently during the session. So, instead of working on the smoking, she was shown how to work on her neck. She noticed an immediate improvement and, by the time she returned two weeks later, her neck was greatly improved and we could then successfully continue with therapy to help her stop smoking.

Hypnosis for pain relief

This is one of the most powerful aspects of hypnotherapy and perhaps also the most controversial. Hypnotic anesthesia was used extensively during surgery in the last century, although those few doctors who did employ it successfully usually risked ridicule and downright hostility from their colleagues.

It is a fact that our bodies can produce their own chemicals to block pain. These are endorphins and enkephalins which share the same chemical properties as morphine. Using hypnosis, we are able to tap into the part of the brain that stimulates the production of these natural painkillers. But, a word of warning: although hypnosis can effectively remove pain, no ethical hypnotherapist would do this type of work without first finding out what was causing the pain. In other words, the client should be asked about the medical diagnosis and the treatment he or she is receiving.

Research over the years has shown that the control of pain occurs not so much through suggestions given by the therapist but rather through the hypnotic state itself. Hypnosis automatically releases endorphins into the bloodstream and enables a dissociation of electrical activities and sensory responses for anaesthesia and analgesia.

One of the areas in which hypnosis can play an important role in providing pain relief is obstetrics. It is a well known fact that tension certainly aggravates, and often causes, pain. So, by helping an expectant mother to relax, by convincing her that she can take control and that childbirth is a completely natural process, we can go halfway towards establishing a state of mind in which she knows that pregnancy and childbirth can be trouble-free. Indeed, childbirth can and should be a joyous occasion, not something that is feared.

A hypnotherapist, who is well trained in advanced methods, should be able to ensure that an expectant mother can go through her pregnancy with relative ease, should be looking forward to the actual birth, and should be able to take complete control of the delivery.

Research into obstetrics over the years has shown that in a large majority of patients using hypnosis, there has been much less need for forceps deliveries, much less need for episiotomies, and that any necessary repair work can be done without chemical anesthetics.

Self-hypnosis

There is really only one effective way to learn self-hypnosis, and that is when you are already in hypnosis. Hence the reason for supplying a hypnotic tape with this book.

An ethical hypnotherapist will automatically teach a client self-hypnosis, usually on the last session, so that the client can then use this gift as a life-enhancing skill for the rest of his life. In this way, he can contact his own subconscious mind, make decisions with the help of the memory banks within his subconscious, program future achievements, and so much more.

Self-hypnosis can of course be used purely for relaxation. Twenty minutes a day spent in a state of mind which automatically recharges one's batteries, which allows the conscious mind to have a rest, and which switches on the parasympathetic nervous system to bring about self-healing within the body, is enormously beneficial.

Self-hypnosis has many advantages over other forms of meditation: it is quicker; it is more directional; and it is safer as it helps you to take complete control over your own mind.

Where to Now
Some questions answered

Having acquired the necessary techniques for taking yourself into self-hypnosis, you may have some queries as to what the next steps should be. Let us have a look at some of those possible questions.

Should I use a cassette recorder?

You may have already decided to record some of the exercises onto a cassette tape—this is certainly a good idea, especially for some of the longer ones.

Perhaps, though, you have doubts about using your own voice on tape—how many of us really like the sound of our own voice? It is best to use your own voice, however, as no one knows better than you what you really want. Rest assured, you will get used to it after a while!

If you do feed suggestions onto tape for yourself to listen to, then you will need to alter our affirmations slightly. You need to speak to yourself as if you were in fact speaking to someone else. For instance, instead of saying "*I am more relaxed*" you should say "*You are more relaxed.*" The subconscious mind accepts suggestions better when they are recorded in this way.

Should I ask a friend to read suggestions to me out loud?

No. Your problems are personal to you. Close as your friend may be, their voice might not be right for you to listen to. In addition, it is worth remembering that one of the major aims of *The Self-Hypnosis Kit* is for you to take responsibility for your own wellbeing. It is also possible that a well-meaning friend might very well try to impose his or her own belief structures on to you.

How long should I stay in hypnosis?

A question that may have come up by now is, "Can I stay in hypnosis for a long period of time?" We have already suggested that a period of around twenty-five minutes once or twice a day is ideal. There are no hard and fast rules to this, except to say that any longer than that would really be too long. It is certainly not our aim to encourage you to withdraw from the world by staying in hypnosis for a long time (pleasant though it is). In fact, as you practice self-hypnosis and the various exercises, you naturally become more confident and therefore more eager to participate in life.

Why can't I change more quickly?

Hopefully by now you will have used at least one of the affirmations in the previous chapter. As we have said before, used on a regular basis, any one of these affirmations should bring about the desired result. If results are a bit slower in coming about than you would want, then just revise the words you are using, perhaps make them more enthusiastic, more specific, or more detailed to your own personal needs. Remember, it is your affirmation—only you know exactly what you desire. And do make sure that you are giving yourself a very clear picture of the way you want yourself to be.

It is important at this stage to be patient with yourself—it has taken you a long time to develop all those old negative habits, so does it really matter if it takes you a few weeks to develop new ones?

Do I really want to change?

This is a big question. The fact is that most of us are frightened of change, so it is just as well at this stage to decide in what areas you genuinely want to make changes—job, health, relationships, finance, spirituality, or whatever.

Having decided on what changes are important to

you, the next step is to provide the commitment to make them happen, to stay with them, and to let the new changes develop into habits. Sometimes even the most negative habits feel comfortable, much like a well-worn article of clothing that has seen better days but fits well. In other words, some habits are hard to discard!

What other books should I read?

Your next choice of reading will probably hinge on why you were interested in our kit in the first place—a general interest in hypnosis and hypnotherapy, or a need to bring about changes within your own persona. There are hundreds of books on hypnosis—some delve into its history, others focus on methods and theory. At the back of this book we list some recommended further reading.

Our Final Message to You

In writing this book we have tried to give you the techniques which will enable you to begin your journey on the road to self-improvement, self-discovery, personal achievement, and enlightenment. In view of the fact that it is not really feasible to provide individual help in a kit, we have tried, as much as possible, to give you tools which are adaptable to suit your needs.

Of course, as with any tool, the more you use it, the more familiar you become with it. You will find that the versatility of the tool increases in direct proportion to your proficiency. So, if at first you do not succeed, then try, try again.

All the techniques we have provided for you have been based on our direct experience of them, as well as our experience in dealing with clients in our private practices, on teaching students in our self-hypnosis and stress management classes, and also on feedback from the hundreds of students we have trained in advanced hypnotherapy. Over the years, these techniques have been altered, honed and adapted, according to the feedback we have received. We therefore acknowledge all those people who have crossed our professional paths and from whom we have learned so much ourselves. Our teaching is based upon the principle of focusing upon the needs of the client, rather than the needs of the therapist, and this principle has been very much kept in mind during the creation of this kit.

We have enjoyed sharing our knowledge with you and would welcome any comments—good or bad. You can write to us at the Corporation of Advanced Hypnotherapy, P.O. Box 70, Southport, PR8 3JB, England.

In the meantime, enjoy the journey.

Further Reading

Chopra, Deepak. *Quantum Healing.* New York: Bantam Books, 1989

Custer, Dan. *The Miracles of Mind Power.* New York: Prentice Hall Press, 1960.

Gawain, Shakti. *Creative Visualization.* New York: Bantam Books, 1979.

Peale, Vincent. *The Power of Positive Thinking.* New York: Prentice Hall Press, 1952.

Peiffer, Vera. *Positively Fearless.* Shaftesbury, England: Element Books, 1993.

Siegel, Bernie, S. Love, *Medicine and Miracles.* London: Arrow Books, 1986.

Index

About the Authors

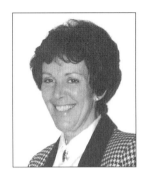

CHERITH POWELL is the Principal of the Atkinson-Ball College of Hypnotherapy and HypnoHealing which specializes in advanced training for hypnotherapists. She runs classes in London and, with her late partner Bill Atkinson-Ball, she has also run workshops in the United States.

She is President of the Corporation of Advanced Hypnotherapy, an elite group of hypnotherapists who have all received postgraduate training. This organization has close links with the British Complementary Medicine Association and has been enthusiastic in lobbying for higher standards and a joint code of ethics for all hypnotherapists in the UK.

Cherith Powell is a member of The British Council of Hypnotist Examiners, The American Council of Hypnotist Examiners, The National Guild of Hypnotists (USA), and The National Federation of Spiritual Healers. She originally trained with Bill Atkinson-Ball but has also studied with many of the top names in hypnotherapy including Ormond McGill, Virginia Satir, Gil Boyne, Ernest Rossi, and Robert Dilts. She has a vast experience in teaching self-hypnosis, having run classes since 1986. She has also run courses in stress management and personal development.

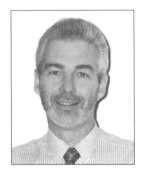

GREG FORDE, an American by birth, first started practicing hypnotherapy in 1967, while in the U.S Forces. Over the years, he developed some of his own hypnotherapy techniques, mainly concerned with rapid inductions and short-term therapy. He first met Bill Atkinson-Ball in 1990 and, after receiving his advanced certificate at the Atkinson-Ball College of Hypnotherapy and HypnoHealing, joined the staff of the college in 1992. He is also Vice-President of the Corporation of Advanced Hypnotherapy, a member of the National Guild of Hypnotists (USA), and a Relate-trained marriage guidance counsellor. He is in private practice in Norfolk, England, regularly giving talks on hypnotherapy as well as running self-hypnosis classes.